The Black Art of Cooking

COPYRIGHT, 1921
by
CARL LOEB, AL D.

Published, September 1921,

COURAGE

For indecision brings its own delays, And days are lost lamenting o'er lost days. Are you in earnest? Seize this very minute What you can do, or dream you can, begin it. Boldness has genius, power and magic in it. Only engage, and then the mind grows heated. Begin, and then the work will be completed.

GOETHE

If you want to know the man who keeps you from accomplishing things; if you want to know what holds you back; if you want to know where to fix the blame, get a looking-glass and look into it carefully.

PREFACE.

It was my endeavor to write a book which is clear and understandable to all, and I hope that I have succeeded.

I did not write this book for the benefit of the profession, but if the few of the profession who after being in practice for years are "still" able to learn something new, they are welcome to any information of value they can find.

This book has been written for the benefit of the maltreated public, to assist them in their study of natures laws, to become free from the oppression of the doctors who displace diseases by introducing worse diseases by means of drugs, serums, vaccines, surgery and maladjustments which is the source of their bread and butter.

I give this book to the public hoping that after reading it they will have less of this destructive, blind faith in doctors, but more real knowledge. As long as there are sick doctors, the public can not have confidence in their knowledge. No more than in a baldheaded barber who sells Hair tonic.

One ounce of knowledge is better than ten pounds of faith."

INDEX

Title—Corrective Feeding—Improper
    Feeding—Definition of Black Art ....   1— 2

How Cooked Food Produces Disease—Natural
    Foods Only Containers of Natural Salts
    —Evidence from Experiments on Animals—Disease Producing Characteristics of Cooked Food—Effects on the
    Windpipe—Lungs— Heart, Large Vein
    —Large Artery—The Liver—The Spleen
    —Esophagus—Stomach— Pyloris, Gallbladder-Small Intestines — Appendix —
    Colon — Rectum—— Piped Colon—
    Appendicitis—Cause of Constipation .....   2—10

Second Part of Evidence—To Seduce Them
    Thru Love Potions—Preparation of Love
    Potions—Love Potions A Sex Stimulant
    —Delicacies—A Cause of Alcoholism —
    Free Lunch—Sexual Over-indulgence—
    Modern Love Potions — Jazz Music—
    Close of Evidence ....   10—15

What is The Proper Food—Why Should We Eat
    Cooked Food—Have Animals Souls—
    College Education—Authority Worship
    —How to Lower the High Cost of
    Living—Wage Workers and their Health
    —Details of Unfired Food—Opposition
    of Wifes — Reasons — Restaurants
    Serving Home Cooked Foods—Why
    Women Oppose the Uncooked Diet—
    Married for Love or Married to a Cook
    —Disadvantages of the Cookpot ....   16—22

Questions answered—Do you eat Grass?—Raw Food— Digestibility of Unfired Food—Authorities and their Mistakes—Which is Easier to Digest?—Faulty Mastication—Eating for Exercise—Fletcherism—Sawdust Experiment—What Indigestion Really is—Fermentation—Paralysis of Stomach and Nerves—Live Food not Fermentable—Is Cooked Food Necessary to Sustain High Reasoning Power—Doctors and Increase of Disease—Modesty in Regard to Disease—Sickness considered a Necessary Experience — Conclusion .... 22—30

How to Begin the Unfired Diet—The Necessary Utensils—Short Fast—Recipes for Beginners .... 30—32

The Psychology of Feeding—Thoughts Alife—The Power of Thought—Your Mentality a Powerful Engine—Control of Mentality—Material Creations of the Mind—Food and Mentality — Concentration — Scientific Eating—The Quick Lunch Room—Penny-wise Businessmen—Illustration—Natural Food not only for the Sick—High Prices and Food—Pluto Water—Warning—Begin Gradually—Reasons for the Thinker—Human Apes—Peppered Fun .... 32—40

Recipes—Health Drinks, their Value—Unfired Lemonade—Orangeade—Herbade—Fruit Frappee—Rhubarbade—Tonic Drink—Near Buttermilk—Lemonized Milk—Unfired Tonic Beer .... 41—44

Soups—Cold or Summer Soups—Pineapple
    Soup—-Cream of Tomato—Panacea—
    Savory—Cranberry and Beet or
    Pumpkin-Banana-Soup .... 44—46

Warm or Winter Soups—Instructions—
    Cranberry Soup— Cream of Celery—
    Banana Cream—Cream of Prune
    Soup: .... 46—47

April Salads—Asparagus—Dandelion—Lentils
    in Nut Cream—Artichoke—Dandelion
    Flower .... 48—49

May Salads—Lettuce and Cocoanut—
    Spinach—Combination—-Radish—
    Linden—Yarrow in Nut Cream—
    Plantain .... 50—51

June Salads—-Lettuce and Cress—Lettuce and
    Parsley—Kohlrabi—Radish and Bean—
    Green Peas in Nut Cream: .... 51—52

July Salads—Stuffed Cantaloupe—Spinach
    Beet—Mock Sauerkraut—Watermelon .... 52—53

August Salads—Tomato and Cucumber
    Sandwiched—-Stuffed Tomato—Sweet
    Corn—Pignolias Potato—Variety—
    Green Tomato and Cress—Squash: —
    Supawn—Ice Plant Salad. .... 54—56

September Salads—Lima Bean and Pumpkin—
    Vege Fruit Salad—Selected Salad—Nut
    Cream Slaw .... 56—57

October Salad—Fall—Artichoke and Sweet Pepper—Kale Selected Salad—Cabbage and Banana—Pea and Cabbage Salad ..... 57—59

Lentils in Honey—Lima Beans in Winter—Simplicity Salads—Banana Relish .... 59—60

Winter Fruit Sauce—Winter Fruit Salad—Mince Fruit— Unfired Poundcake—Pie Fillings—Apple Cream Pie—Prune or Plum Pie Apple and Banana Pie— Banana Mousse—Mixed Fruit Sauce .... 60—63

Illustrations—Crepe Hangers Hymn—Photo of the Author 64

Meat—Fat and Protein—Nuts Better Substitutes—What Meat is—Reasonable Priced Meat—Past of an Appetizing Stake—Your Stomach Knows—Meat and Hard Work—Prof. Voits Findings—Other Evidence —The Kuli — The Icelanders —Prevalence of Disease—Overconsumption of Protein—Results—Contents of Meat—Comparison—Albumen Poisoning—How to Build a Home for Scavengers—Is Chicken and Fish Meat?—Soup—-Meat Containing Animal Magnetism—The Grave of Dead Animals .... 65—69

Cereals—Hard to Digest—Bread—"Poor Food"—The Yeast Fake 70

THE BLACK ART OF COOKING — xi

Sugar a Disease Producer—Candy—Cause of
Malnutrition—Sugar a Strong Irritant—
Mashproducer—Experiment on Natures
Sugar—Advertising Schemes—Grape
Sugar—Cocoa and Chocolate—Death
Rate in Sugar Factories .... 71—73

Salt—A Habit—Salt Covers Filthy Conditions—
Observations made by Dr. Stephanson—
Diseases Caused by Salt—Defense—Old
Age—Non-assimilation .... 74—75

Milk—Food for Calves — Pasteurization —
Milking Un natural—Sanitary Humbug
— Lemonized Milk—Milk Cures A
Fad—Butter—Cottage Cheese—Poem—
Constipation of the Brain .... 76—78

Menstruation—A Natural Function—Unfired
Diet Regulating the Flow 79

Venereal Diseases—Cause—Uselessness of
Serum etc.—Laboratory Tests
Unreliable—Example—Failure of the
Microscopic Test—Results—You Need
an Operation—Germs are Symptoms
not Causes—One Reliable Test—The
Inventor—Description of the B. D. C.
Test—Women Protect Your Future—All
Disease Curable—Unfired Food Cures
Venereal Diseases .... 79—84

Food in Relation to Sex—Sex not Sinful—The
Sexual Instinct—A Mistake of the
Creator—Ascetics Mostly Weaklings—
Conditions Necessary for a Happy

Marital Union—Marriage Licenses do not Create Happiness—Sex a Product of the Mind—Cooked Food Un balances the Mind—Effect of Foods Stimulation—Food that Energizes Sex — False Ideas—Sex Instruction—Innocence not a virtue .. 85—88

The Action of the Heart and Kidneys in the Unfired Diet—Saving of the Heart—Gravity of Urine—Result— Weight .... 89—90

The Starving Babies of America .... 91—95

The First Telegraph System—A Little Story for Big Children .... 97—101

Dear Reader—Apyrtrophism Not a Fad—Warning—The Apyrtropher Society—The Apyrtropher Magazine—Write for Sample—Finis .... 101—102

THE BLACK ART OF COOKING

The title of this book may not create much sympathy for the author among some of the readers of the "fair" sex who take pleasure in preparing over the cook stove many complex articles of food for their bountiful table and who feel proud of their ability to tickle the most fastidious palate. But the author is well aware of the chances he is taking when he "sticks his nose" into milady's kitchen and shows "so little respect" for the intricate science of cooking. He can see in his mental picture "the turned up noses and scornful glances" of the experts of the cookpot, saying, "The Black Art of Cooking—why—what do you mean, sir?"

The members of the opposite sex, in getting interested, will say "Come on, boys, he's started something! Let's watch the rumpus."

The writer does not underestimate the strength of his opponents when it comes to battles fought with words and brains, but he is well prepared and ready to let the bystanders be the judges. Experience has taught him that sometimes those who oppose him most at first become his best friends later on and appreciate the bigger life in store for them, with greater happiness, more time to do those things the inner woman craves, greater health, less fatigue, and a greater chance to enjoy heaven on earth. They have also found that friend husband was less irritable, worked harder, made more money, and that the children missed their usual sickness, made better grades at school, and that the family doctor's bills were shattered.

In the end woman finds that the author has really deeply appreciated her situation and wants to lend his best aid in making woman's dream of idealism come true.

Corrective feeding is one of the most vital subjects of the day, because man is made up of what is put into him, just the same as a building is made up of the material placed in it. Every vital organ, every nerve, every bone, every muscle, every ligament and every cell in the body requires certain food elements to make them function properly, and this is only possible with proper food.

Dr. John H. Tilden sums it up nicely when he says, "There is nothing with which man has to do that is of more importance than a knowledge of food, its composition, preparation, and effect upon the body; its good as well as bad effects, its conversion into brain and brawn." For it has all to do with health, and without health nothing can be accomplished."

Improper feeding leaves a trail of woe behind. So with this in mind the writer "sticks his nose into the kitchen" and talks about "The Black Art."

Marquart in his work, "The Religion of the Romans" gives the following definition of "Black Art": "The main purposes of the black art or black magic are: to harm the good (healthy) whenever possible by creating disease, insanity or death, to seduce them through love potions by summoning the dead and spirits of vengeance, and to use the knowledge of their art to harm humanity in every way possible."

Since cooking is called a "Black Art" by the author, let us see whether this assertion can be justified in accordance with the definition given above.

First: "To harm the good (healthy) whenever possible by creating disease, insanity or death"

HOW COOKED FOOD PRODUCES DISEASE.

The process of applying fire or heat to food for a certain length of time is called cooking. There are a variety of ways in which fire or heat is applied to food. Sometimes it is applied directly, but more often indirectly through pots or pans. These dishes usually contain fat or water which is brought to a high temperature and the food to be cooked is immersed in the contents of the dish. We are not interested in the different ways of cooking but we want to know what happens to the food when it goes through the process of cooking.

The application of fire or heat to anything for a length of time will change this particular thing.

What this change is which takes place in food by the application of heat is a vital thing to know.

All natural foods are containers of salts in natural biologic combinations. These natural combinations are known under the terms of vitamins It is impossible to live without these organized salts or vitamins. When one cooks these containers of organized salts, they disorganize the salts, and they cease to be that which one could properly call "food".

The superficial chemist denies the above statements because he has failed to find a way to test the fundamental differences, but the stomach, the intestines, the liver, the pancreas, the salivary glands, the thyroid gland, the nerves and kidneys suffer from that difference and in consequence each cell throughout the body suffers from that difference. Since it is not possible to prove this through chemical analysis, it is necessary to produce better evidence, such as results, from the following experiments:

1. Sheep fed entirely oil cooked food died within five months.
2. Eight hogs were experimented on. Four of them were fed on cooked food and four were given an uncooked diet. The four fed the strict cooked food died within six months of the cholera, the other four even though they came in contact with the diseased hogs were immune, and are still alive.
3. Mice fed entirely on white bread died sooner than mice that did not get any food. It has generally

been found that animals fed on cooked food are more susceptible to disease than animals living on natural food. Monkeys in captivity that are fed on cooked food easily die of consumption. Hagenbeck, the well known animal trainer, has never found a case of consumption among any of his monkeys fed strictly on natural food. Such circumstances would certainly lead one to believe that there is a difference in cooked food and natural food even though it cannot be analyzed by present day chemical analysis such as is usually employed. If the same food produces disease when it is cooked and in its natural state prevents disease, as is shown in the case of the hogs with cholera, then there MUST be a radical difference between cooked and uncooked food.

If this contention be true, humans who live mostly on cooked food ought to be suffering more of disease than the animal that lives on natural food. They must be also more susceptible to infectious diseases. Furthermore, if natural food tends to prevent disease in animals, it must also give humans the same immunity.

The disease producing characteristic of cooked food can be expressed as follows:
1. Hypersolubility of the starches and proteins, resulting in hypersaturation of the blood with undesirable food material which becomes a useless burden and finally a poison.
2. Disarrangement of the atoms in the organic molecule of all food-material when cooked which may be expressed as follows; cooked sugar has become inorganic sugar; cooked starch has become inorganic starch; cooked protein has become inorganic protein; cooked organic salts have become inorganic salts.
3. Extreme fermentability of the starchy as well as the proteid food.

Furthermore, the bacteria active in food fermentation produce a more virulently toxic waste from cooked food than from natural food, which rarely occurs in the latter.

This is proven by the fact that when cooked food ferments it may only stimulate the nerves controlling the peristaltic muscles, resulting in constipation; whereas when natural food ferments it may only stimulate the peristaltic functions, resulting in laxation.

It should not be forgotten, however that the toxic product of fermenting cooked food is not limited to paralyzing the nerves of peristalsis but that it also penetrates to the nerves of the heart, the lungs, the liver, the pancreas, the kidneys and especially the organs of procreation, which lie in closest proximity; first irritating them, then perverting them and finally paralyzing them.

So far cooking has proven to be Black Art in the fullest sense of the word, now let us see what cooked food does to the different organs. (The illustration of the different organs as found in "Un-fired Food and Trophotheraphy" borrowed by courtesy of the author.)

1. **Windpipe** (Trachea). Here is where the inorganic product of cooked starch and cooked sugar together with some table salt and other unorganized salts, absorbed from cooked food, are often eliminated in the form of catarrh accompanied by inflammation. Should the bacillus tuberculosis find its way into these tissues while burdened with the filth the catarrh may turn into consumption.

2,2 **The Lungs**. When the product of cooked carbohydrates (inorganic sugar and starch) accumulate in the tissues of the lungs and is eliminated into the bronchioles, it is called catarrh of the lungs. When the mucous fluid containing this filth cannot be exhaled, it becomes destructive to the lung-tissues.

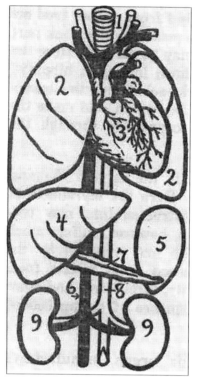

When the bacillus tuberculosis finds its way into this morbid accumulation, causing wholesale destruction of the lungs, it is called consumption.

3. **The Heart   6. The Large Vein.   8. Large Artery** These are the vessels into which the undesirable material absorbed from cooked food accumulates and becomes a poison to any weak part of the body to which it may be carried. Here the cooked protein breaks down into uric, hippuric, sulphuric and phosporic acids and the carbohydrates into carbonic acid, which acid make the blood so viscid that it cannot go through the capillaries (hair veins).

4. **The Liver.** This is the largest chemical laboratory of the body. Here the byproducts of natural food are reconstructed into new useful elements. This organ, however, suffers much from being clogged with and irritated by the inorganic material absorbed from cooked food. Here congestion, inactivity, torpid liver and other liver trouble are the sequence of eating cooked food.

5. **The Spleen.** This organ manufactures and replenishes good blood from Natural Food; but cooked food may be so devoid of material to convert into good blood that anaemia (want of good blood) may follow.

The Black Art of Cooking

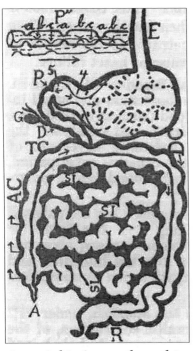

E Esophagus. S Stomach. P Pyloris. The lines 1, 2, 3, and 4 represent the successive, progressive peristaltic contractions. The arrows at 2, 3 and 4 show how the food churns back through the neck of the contraction until it becomes ripe to pass through the pyloris at P., indicated by the arrow under 5. The function of the sphincter muscles of the pyloris is not to relax until the acid gastric juice is neutralized on proteid food; but when food ferments it generates more acid than can be neutralized and the irritation of this keeps the sphincter muscles tense, so that no food can pass. Cooked starchy food is extremely apt to ferment in the stomach and when it does ferment the volatile acid produced paralyzes the nerves that control the peristaltic contractions 1,2,3 and 4 and often this paralyzing influence penetrates to the solar plexus. This when temporary is called acute indigestion and when it is persistent it is called chronic indigestion. The acid and alcohol absorbed from the fermenting food is what finally produces that craving for whiskey and other fermented drinks. Thus, cooked food is the link between the kitchen and the saloon. When the autointoxication penetrates to the nerves of the heart it may be the cause of heart failure.

D Duodenum, G Gall Bladder. SI, SI and SI. Small Intestines, In the duodenum and small intestines cooked proteid food (such as cooked peas, and baked beans) ferments and paralyzes the nerves that control the peristaltic movements of the intestines, which is the cause of constipation. The fermentation of cooked proteid food is generally indicated by flatulency.

Sometimes when the stomach has been abused by fermentation for a long time the sphincter muscles of the pyloris become lax and allow the fermenting food to pass into the intestines and thus also causing constipation and autointoxication.

The diagram above the stomach, under "P" illustrates how the peristaltic contraction, of the intestines, under a, a, a progresses to b, b, b, and then to c, c, c.

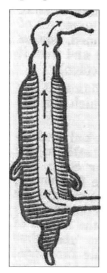

A Appendix. A C Ascending Colon. D C Descending Colon. R Rectum. Albuminous food (flesh and eggs) ferments and decays in the ascending colon and there paralyzes the nerves that control the peristaltic contractions, indicated by the arrows under A C.

When the muscles of the ascending colon are relaxed by the toxins produced by fermentation then the colon fills like a bag (see "Piped Colon") and the moisture next to the wall of the colon is absorbed, thereby making a rigid wall of food (indicated by the shaded area). Inside of the rigid pipe, the food still remains flexible and soft and this portion is forced upward (see arrows) by the pressure of food coming from the intestines.

When the colon has been piped for a long time then the typhoid germ makes its home between the hard pipe and the wall of the colon.

Where the typhoid germ colonizes it produces irritating waste which forms abscesses in the wall of the colon. These abscesses finally become lateral appendixes, giving much pain.

Many surgeons in their wise ignorance offer to clip the terminal or natural appendix A, ("which really produces a lubricant for the colon") saying that then the patient can not develop appendicitis and that it is a useless organ anyway. The illustration shows that this is not true and it is proven that nine cases out of ten are of the lateral kind. When the typhoid germ colonizes at the mouth of the appendix this organ becomes inflamed, relaxes and allows morbid food to fall into it and then it may be called appendicitis (see piped colon).

As long as the appendix is not inflamed it has a powerful peristaltic contraction which can lift any foreign body out of its mouth.

The toxic effect of fermented cooked food increases as it passes through the intestines, the ascending, transverse and descending colon and rectum. It stands to reason, that the fermenting food which paralyzes the nerves that control the peristaltic contractions; (causing constipation) will also have the same influence on the nerves of all the vital organs that are in the abdominal cavity, paralyzing or perverting their functions; thus, giving rise to all abdominal troubles. This makes plain, how many female troubles have their origin in the autointoxication (self poisoning) of fermenting cooked food. Since autointoxication causes the food to move extremely slowly through the colon, there is too much time given to the absorption of its moisture and hence it becomes very hard feces as it enters the rectum. These hard feces, then, mechanically break the layers of muscles that cover the rectum from one another. The breaks thus produced fill with blood like a blister making piles and hemorrhoids. The blood in the piles becomes fetid from the toxic feces and is converted into puss which eats its way into the rectal cavity and discharges.

It is well known that the flatus, passed by those who do not eat meat, is but slightly offensive; whereas the flatus, passed by those who feed on natural food, is almost always imperceptible.

The scientific world has hitherto overlooked the fact that nascent acid, newly produced by acid fermentation and nascent alcohol newly produced by alcoholic fermentation, are vastly more toxic and paralyzing to the nerve tissues than acids and alcohols which have become stale or settled as such. In other words—a mere trace of nascent acid in the contents of the alimentary canal paralyzes the nerves more effectively than a sip of comparatively stale, but pure vinegar. To illustrate— Everybody has experienced that fresh milk which ferments in the stomach and intestines constipates; whereas clabbered milk in which the acid is stale, only stimulates a defensive peristaltic activity and this is the source of its laxative property. Upon these facts hinges the whole subject of autointoxication.

The above is ample proof that the first part of the contention that cooked food produces disease, insanity and finally death, is correct. Therefore cooked food fulfills the first three purposes of "Black Art", as defined above: To harm the good (healthy) whenever possible by creating disease, insanity, or death.

Let us see further whether the contention that cooking is A BLACK ART is correct.

"TO SEDUCE THEM THROUGH LOVE POTIONS"

In olden times, old women of ill-repute, known as witches, used to brew "love potions." These potions were supposed to have the power to create love for the possessor by mixing a few drops of the potion in the food or drink of the person to be seduced.

Under the cover of night when all the world was asleep, men and women would sneak to the hut of the witch who usually lived alone in some secluded spot in the woods with her cats, skulls, crossbones and other paraphernalia which was necessary to hoodwink the public

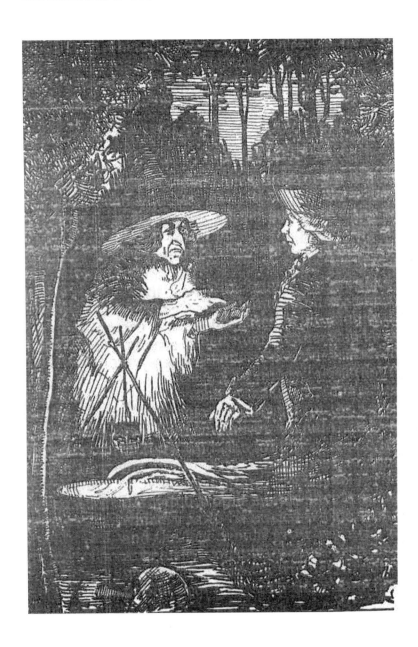

of the past just like the quacks of today who use germs, serum and magic terms for diseases. (See page 15)

The consultant would tell the witch his motives and she would give advice according to the ability of the pocketbook of the consultant. In case the consultant was a poor farmer or herd girl, the witch would simply give a little root or twig which was to be buried with a lock of the beloved, and the love would grow with the root. But when a wealthy consultant appeared on horseback the witch would brew a wonderful potion. Such a love potion required some hair and fingernails of the horseman. The witch would take the skull and crossbones from the shelf and draw magic circles with the crossbones around the fire over which hung a boiling kettle filled with herbs, roots, spiders, snakes and other similar ingredients. She would then ride around the fire on her broomstick, then add the hair and nails of the consultant to the mixture while mumbling strange words and terms to the trembling consultant, such as tonsillitis, high blood pressure, low blood pressure, colitis, procitis, eczema, bacillus and like words, the only essential being that the consultant could remember the terms used. I do not know whether the witch used the same terms that I have used above but if she was a modern up-to-date witch she would use them because they have proven to be very successful and will always create a great deal of admiration and respect among the "trade" who marvel at the person who knows and is able to pronounce such "hard" words.

Then the potion would be poured into a container which was delivered to the contestant with very complicated instructions, when, how and where to use the potion. The consultant left relieved of his sorrow and his money. If the potion did the work, the witch got plenty of free advertising; if it did not work, the consultant was informed that he did not follow the directions correctly, and he needed another potion, provided he was willing or able to pay for it. Just like today, the operation was not successful—you need another operation.

We are getting away from our subject; what has this all to do with cooking? How does cooked food represent a love potion and how does it seduce ?

At first sight the word "love potion" seems quite harmless, because we associate all good with "love", but if we investigate we find another wolf in sheep's clothing.

While the intentions of the person who administered a love potion to a member of the opposite sex, may have often been very good, the means innocently used were always evil. All love potions were bad and always harmful, because they never created love but if they were effective they always acted as a sex stimulant.

Sex, the highest function in all life, is changed into the most destructive and evil function, when stimulated into action by anything but love.

While cooked food is not consciously employed as a sex stimulant today, we know that all feasts in the past have ended with orgies of tremendous proportions. You will answer that cooked food did not cause these orgies, but fermented liquids, like ale, awa, met, wine, beer, whisky, etc. I admit this point but the food was prepared and seasoned in such a manner that it caused a great desire for drinking, furthermore it must not be forgotten that the large quantities of cooked food in the stomach of the participants at the feast, underwent a process of fermentation, and the alcohol produced in the stomach is more powerful and destructive than any ordinary alcoholic drink.

Today we have arrived at a point of perversion where we pay exorbitant prices for food prepared by a person who has made a specialty of compounding mixtures, to tickle (stimulate) the human palate. When a cook is able to tickle the palate of his victims successfully he receives the title chef, and his creations become "delicacies." Some time ago the press brought the announcement that the chef of a certain New York Hotel (I am not going to mention the name because I do not get paid for advertising, like the press which brings or suppresses news when paid for), draws a salary of $50,000 per year. If this hotel is paying $50,000 for stimulating the palates of the victims into over-indulgence in food and drink, it must receive at least 3 to 4 times of this amount in return in the business of selling cooked food which produces disease and many other evils.

All cooked delicacies have one common effect: they confuse the nerves of the tongue palate and stomach in a way that those nerves are unable to determine when the system has the proper amount of food, or in other words, cooked highly seasoned foods are responsible for a great deal of alcoholism. While we had saloons they were able to give a free lunch to their patrons because this free lunch was only free to the saloonkeeper, for the victim usually paid for it in alcoholic drinks. When our saloons went "dry" the free lunch had to be paid for by the saloonkeeper and it disappeared. Another case where cooked food has proven to be a Black Art.

The orgies of today therefore have the same foundation as those of the past. A prominent medical writer said: "We are suffering at present more from over-eating and over-indulgence in sex than of any other cause." I say, we only suffer from over-eating. Sexual over-indulgence is simply a symptom of over-eating of cooked food.

Here is where the love potion comes in. This is the composition of a present-day love potion. Stimulation by sensual inartistic imitations of music, known under the term of "jazz', suggestive dancing and suggestive dress, which is not caused by exposure but by camouflaging and partly exposing the natural form. After the dance comes a little dinner party, consisting of combinations of intricately seasoned foods which stimulate the nerves causing an abnormal appetite for food and especially alcoholic drinks. Over-eating causes fatigue as we can see by the fat man who always wants to sleep when he is not eating. Fatigue is caused by accumulation of waste in the system; this waste blurs the judgment and with the help of the alcohol caused by internal fermentation of the food, and the addition of the alcoholic drinks demanded by an over-stimulated system, the resistance and reasoning power of the victim is lowered to such a degree, that it is an easy prey to the seducer.

That all the other contentions of Black Art are true is self-evident; a person with the reasoning power lowered by over-stimulation through cooked food and its effect (alcohol) will easily arouse the spirits of vengeance which are powerless in the normal state of a person, and harm himself and humanity in general.

This concludes the evidence against cooked food. I am satisfied to justly call cooking a Black Art, and that I have proven that cooked food harms the good (healthy), by creating disease, insanity and death. That cooked food seduces like a "love potion." That cooked food is responsible for many crimes of vengeance and summons the dead powers of evil in a person, which are brought to life and into action by autointoxication caused by cooked food.

Finally that the knowledge of said art of cooking is used to harm humanity in every way possible, therefore this art must rightfully be classed as

A BLACK ART.

I have shown the various faults of cooked food and I have proven that it is neither beneficial nor wholesome, therefore it is not the proper food for the human animal.

WHAT IS THE PROPER FOOD?

Uncooked, unfired, natural food, as prepared (cooked) by nature, is the only correct food for man. I will prove to you that this contention is correct if you will give me your whole attention.

I am in the same position as the man who was asked to prove why we should sleep in a reclining position, instead in a standing one. If you were in that man's position you would say: "why don't you prove to me first, why a man should sleep in a standing position?"

Why should we eat cooked food? We are the only members of the animal kingdom who eat cooked food. There is no reason why we should be different from the animal and eat cooked food. You may say that we are different in many respects; for instance, we can use our reason when we are speaking and laughing. These two methods of expression are the only differences between the human and the animal. We have a soul. If we have, this same law must hold good with all living organisms. Some may deny that an animal has reason. I believe that animals can reason, and anyone who has studied animals will admit that. Even if we admit that we are superior in some faculties than all the other animals, we are simply in a class for ourselves in certain faculties, i.e., we are the highest developed animal in regard to reasoning power, and that is all, and no more.

It is often necessary to start an argument about something to get people interested. I started an argument about cooked food, to awaken some interest, to get the people to think. Thinking has become an automatic art in our modern days of civilization (?). Most of us have forgotten to think independently. For the common man the press does the thinking. For the college man who received an automatic education, the "authority" does the thinking. The common man will often think independently and act according to his own ideas. But our "educated" class will mostly bow to the opinion of their authorities. If a great authority pronounces a disease incurable, the patient if "educated" (i. e. college-educated to respect authorities), will invariably go home and await death. He does not dare to think that authorities are human and products of circumstances, that they are able to make mistakes. But patients pronounced "incurable", by some of the greatest authorities, have been cured, and have visited the graves of these great authorities.

I hope, I awakened some of you, who usually put their mind under the influence of some "ossified" authority, and think according to the authorities suggestion.

Are you awake? Consider me an authority, ossified, whiskered, with high self-esteem who thinks "I am always right and I can force my opinion on you, because I know you dare not challenge me."

If I woke you up, you will challenge every statement I make and try to refute it; if you can not refute it, you can give me credit; but do not think, because I have been right this time, that I am unable to make a mistake the next time. Keep on fighting and you will protect yourself from illusions, and you will do me a great favor by protecting me from self-esteem and ossification.

We took a walk and got away from our subject, let us get back to it, quickly. I said, Uncooked, Unfired Natural Food as prepared (cooked) by nature is the only correct food for man. I will now explain the practice of Unfired feeding. Before I begin I can save some of the readers time. If you are of the type of reader who does not have to eat Unfired Food, because you are not sick, kindly put this book away until you are sick. If you are situated so that the high cost of living does not affect you and you do not necessarily have to depend on your two hands to support your person and your family, the following may not be worth while for you, dear reader. I do not think it is necessary for me to warn the fatties of both sexes, who's greatest enjoyment and purpose in life is Eating, Drinking and Sleeping and excessive living in general, because they are not going to read this book. They have no "time" to read, except occasionally the newspaper, if they don't fall asleep over it.

I am trying to show you, working men and women, how you can improve the present conditions under which you are existing, and how you can lower the high cost of living and at the same time raise the standard of your health as well as of your families.

The wage workers' existence depends entirely on the state of their health, because the only commodity they have to sell is their labor. It is of the greatest importance for you to know how you can keep your body in a condition, so it is able to produce this commodity for the longest possible time. Some of the readers may feel offended because I speak about the human body like one would about a piece of machinery; but the human body is a machine and the body of the wageworker is treated as such. If this machine of the worker does not function properly at top speed, it is discarded, or in commercial terms, "he is kicked out", and instantly replaced by a newer (younger) machine. These human machines are so plentiful and replaced at such a low cost, that it does not even pay the owner of such a machine to have it repaired, in most cases it is simply thrown on the human junk pile.

The foregoing reasons, I think, are sufficient to make the average worker who is able to think, sit up and take notice. The subject under consideration is so unusual that it takes some preliminary explanations before approaching it. Because our parents and grand parents have eaten cooked food all their life, is no reason to discard the idea of unfired food, no more than such a reason would keep you from riding in an automobile or airship, if the opportunity presented itself.

The Black Art of Cooking 19

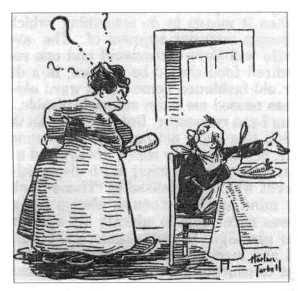

But how about the details of this system. Must one discard the frying pan, the cook-stove and the kitchen and simply have a little pantry with a few dishes for serving the meals and for storing food?

Here we are coming to the greatest stumbling-stone of the unfired system, the "Black Artist" in person, friend 'wifey' the cook. Very often a man can see the necessity and value of the unfired diet, and he presents the unfired idea to his better half, who very often proves to be his worst halt especially when it means to do something which the other people may not approve of. The average housewife will have a thousand and one reasons why unfired food should be tabooed, in a decent, regular old-fashioned home. This word old-fashioned has caused me more stomach trouble, than anything I can remember. Before I went on the unfired diet, this word old-fashioned, in connection with pie, beans, soup or stews, always had a magnetic attraction on my mind when displayed in a restaurant which specialized in "Home Cooking", but my mind and my stomach always disagreed, and I was never able to educate my stomach, to consider nice signs in restaurants, and beautifully colored and nicely flavored foods. I surely tried my best to educate this ignorant (?) stomach, to "home made", "old-fashioned", "just like mother made it", etc., foods, without avail. The cost of this campaign of education was my appendix and nearly my life. Since I have adopted the unfired diet, my mind and stomach are a very happy couple and agree on all food questions.

Most of the members of the "stronger" sex will continue to live the "old-fashioned" way, and never attempt to raise the unfired food question again and would rather suffer heroically from the effects of cooked food than argue the question with friend 'wifey', the cook. The trouble with the members of the "stronger" sex is that they are physically stronger than the women, but mentally weaker than the weaker sex; because they can be appeased by any unfounded argument when it comes from friend wife.

There is another reason for the enmity, the average woman has to unfired food. This fundamental reason she wisely never puts in the field of argument. This is another sign of mental superiority of the weaker sex.

I shall be indiscrete enough to give this fundamental reason. It takes much time, experimenting and burned fingers to acquire the "Black Art of Cooking" It takes practice to kill food by burning it just enough to be cooked, without carrying this process of destruction to -the point where the dead food tastes burned. Do you blame a woman when she fights to retain this practice she took so much pains to acquire, and in many instances the first and last "Art" many women will ever master, because between the cookpot, the washtub, and the offspring most women cannot find time to learn and grow mentally, they are forced to stand still "Die Liebe geht durch den Magen" (Love appeals thru the stomach), is an old German proverb, and like most old things, out of date. The woman of today wants to be more than her husband's servant This proverb came down from the days when man looked down on the female as a piece of property owned by him, but inferior to himself. The woman of today, the real woman, wants a partner, a mate and companion; not a person whose selfish love is based on the black art of cooking. The man who loves a woman for her ability to cook is usually loved by this woman for his ability to provide for her. Some people call this love; I call it business.

When a man is married to his cook, he usually has a sweetheart besides, and his man-friends are his companions. He can only be found at home when he eats or sleeps. Can you blame him for not staying at home? A woman that can only cook can not entertain him, except with neighbors' back-porch gossip. For such a woman a man who works regularly, brings home his pay, likes her cooking, "licks" the children when necessary, and takes her to visit neighbors or relatives twice a year, is considered a good husband.

Suppose a woman sees that she is losing ground, that she is unable to hold her husband's love with the cookpot; when she tries to take interest in her husbands world and begins to study she finds that cooking takes up so much time daily that she is unable to spend any time for her mental growth. Her brain becomes dormant and useless for anything except gossip and "what'll I cook today?"

Even if married life is not built up on a mutual "business proposition" and the foundation is real love, this love can not last unless both partners grow together. After marriage the woman is mostly confined behind the cook stove, preparing meals for hours, which are devoured in a few minutes. The man, being outside, sees and hears, his ideas and interests change; his partner, his sweetheart and wife, stands still, her ideas are the same as those when the married life began. The man can not find anymore interest in conversation with the woman who was his only interest a little while ago, he has outgrown her, they lost one another because he grew and she stood still. The great tragedy of married life. Two strangers living together in one home with different ideas and ideals, a tragedy caused by the cookpot.

If it was not for the cookpot, mothers could be the playmates of their children and would be considered their friends, instead of being classed among such worries as school teachers, home work, policemen and enemies of all fun.

If it was not for the cookpot, husbands and wives would be pals all the time; their interest would be common and a man would not have to feel that he could not bring his wife along to the club because she is a woman and all the other "fellers" would feel embarrassed because a woman is around, claiming women, "especially married ones", are so "silly and monotonous", always talking about clothes and food.

Can you see the great disadvantage of the cookpot?

Perhaps I have made some enemies, but the cookpot has made more, and I believe it is worth the price I may have paid in friendships.

QUESTIONS ANSWERED.

"You do not eat meat or anything cooked, well what do you eat; raw potatoes or grass"?, is a common question asked.

The Apyrtropher (Unfired Fooder) does not eat anything "Raw". Most people do not really know what raw food is. The common idea is that uncooked food is raw food. Did you ever consider that the cook needs this so-called raw food to beautify his "unnatural foods", using parsley, lettuce, radishes, etc., for trimming?

Unfired Food is the most aesthetic and tasty of all foods and if prepared according to the directions given in this book, the reader will have a treat in store.

For those who like to try some RAW food, I would advise them to eat some half-grown sour apples, quarter-grown tomatoes, unripe persimmons, dandelion roots or oysterplant-roots. Try any of these and you will learn what "Raw" food is. The Apyrtropher System (Unfired Food System) also holds that all cooked food is irredeemably "raw", by being made fit for the "scavenger yeast-germ", because the product of this germ paralyzes the functional nerves of digestion.

The digestibility of Unfired Food is questioned very often by the average person. Many authorities (?) even hold that unfired food is indigestible and should not be given to people with digestive troubles. But in spite of these statements by authorities we are not only giving unfired food to patients with poor digestion but we are using this very unfired, indigestible (?) food to relieve the diseased condition of the patient, and in most cases this mode of diet will cure the most obstinate cases of Indigestion, which could not even have been relieved by any other kind of treatment. Think!

The following I quote from the Food Reformers Year Book of 1921, published by the Vegetarian Society of London; it will give the reader a good idea of the misinformation prevalent in regard to digestion and unfired food.

NON-COOKED FOOD.

By F. Stevenson Hooker, MD., L.R.CP., L. R. C. S.

Many and interminable discussions are now taking place between the advocates of a cooked diet and a raw one. It may be said at once that if health alone be considered, it could be maintained, and that perhaps very thoroughly, on the so-called uncooked diet, while of course much valuable time would be saved, to say nothing of firing and in cook's wages, etc. On the other hand, a very large percentage of the people are wanting in perfect digestion, and these certainly would not expect to do well on a raw dietary."

In the Apyrtropher Magazine of July 1921, Dr. Geo. J. Drews answered Dr. Hooker's statement. The article will answer questions in regard to the digestibility of Unfired Food.

WHICH IS EASIER TO DIGEST?

On account of the misinterpretation of the words "digestible" and "indigestible" the people are misled into wrong ideas of food and wrong selections of food with the consequences of suffering and disease beyond local stomach troubles.

To come closer to a common understanding let us quote from Webster:

"**Digest**—To separate the food in its passage through the alimentary canal into the nutritive and non-nutritive elements; to prepare, by the action of the digestive juices, for conversion into chyme."

"**Digestion**—The conversion of food, in the stomach and intestines, into soluble and diffusible products, capable of being absorbed by the blood."

"**Indigestion**—A failure of the normal (chemical) changes which food should undergo in the alimentary canal"

"**Indigestible**—Not readily soluble in the digestive juices; not easily convertible into products fitted for absorption."

From these definitions some people come to the conclusion that all the food ingested is digested, i. e. becomes nutrition. This is not true. Digestion is only a process of separating the soluble nutritive elements from the fiber and insoluble elements. The stomach and intestines have no teeth for comminution; but if fiber and other insoluble matter could be reduced to minute particles, that would not make them absorbable, nor diffusible nor useful in the bloodstream as nutrition.

Cooking breaks up some of the looser fiber and cellulose; but does not make them more digestible to the stomach or intestines and in cases where they are boiled under high pressure so that these particles become soluble enough to enter into the blood stream, they are then the more indigestible to the individual cells that are hungry.

Now because cooking breaks up some of the fiber and cellulose and thus makes an even mass of the food, no matter how poorly it is masticated, the chunks and pieces do not show in the stools. This makes some people think that such products have been properly digested when on the contrary this state has nothing to do with the chemistry of digestion. When these same people eat unfired food from which the nutritive elements are more easily extracted and separated and absorbed, but because of their faulty mastication, chunks and pieces show up in the stools, they are at once alarmed and frightened over the indigestibility of the unfired food.

Strawberry seeds, blackberry seeds, apple seeds and grape seeds are absolutely indigestible and all of them germinate and grow when they are deposited in the stools along the country hedge. This causes no alarm whatever, but if a piece of celery, a piece of uncooked asparagus, a piece of cucumber, a piece of cabbage, a piece of apple skin, a half of a wheat berry or a chunk of a nut were found in the stools digestion would be blamed at once with fear of stomach trouble.

One stingy woman was disappointed over the wastefulness of unfired food when she found some unmasticated pieces of apple in the alvine deposits and because the unfired food did not constipate her she thought that she did not get her money's worth out of that food.

One man could hardly believe it when we told him that less than an ounce of nutritive substance is digested and absorbed into the bloodstream out of a full meal irrespective of the weight of the food eaten. Less than a half of an ounce of proteid material is absorbed for the repair of various tissues and the remainder is in the form of sugar which is used up for heat and energy. Honey does not require digestive action and therefore as much as four ounces may be absorbed and burnt up for heat and energy without detrimental consequences; however, this amount is not required for the maintenance of health.

Most of the food eaten is, therefore, required to exercise the alimentary nerves and muscles. To reduce the quantity of food required by excessive mastication is not desirable, because of the deterioration and dwindling of the alimentary nerves and muscles for want of exercise. Fletcher succeeded in maintaining health on cooked food by chewing everything to absolute liquidity; but he could have lived twice as long, at least, if he would have developed strong alimentary nerves and muscles by eating unfired food as Nature intended.

In one of our public lectures we demonstrated that an absolutely indigestible fiber, such as linden sawdust, did not interfere with the process of digestion. To impress the audience with the truth of the fact, right there before their eyes we combined two ounces of chopped lettuce, one ounce of shredded carrots and two ounces of shredded cucumber, and one ounce of flaked nuts. Then we added three heaping teaspoonsful of the sawdust and a teaspoon of honey and stirred the whole together and proceeded to eat this sawdust synede to the finish. Then we went on to tell them that this sawdust would exercise the intestines, sweep them clean, stimulate peristalsis and absorb poisons that are thrown into the intestinal canal to be carried out

The indigestion that the world of patients complains of is not due to the indigestibility of the food. The secret and truth of it is this: All cooked food is subject to yeast invasion in the stomach. When the product of the yeast fermentation (alcohol) paralyzes the nerves of the stomach and intestines then the digestive process stops together with the muscular movements and then they call it indigestion. It is true—this is indigestion; but it is not due to the indigestibility of food. It is due to the food being predigested and thus made ready for the yeast invasion. The yeast is a scavenger and it only invades dead semi-liquid or liquid food, such as cooked food becomes in the stomach.

The fermentation of a combination of both cooked and sweet unfired food causes a consternation worse than that described above. It may not only paralyze the nerves of the stomach, but headache and nausea may follow. Where a still larger variety is mixed in the stomach at one sitting and the stomach still holding an active yeast from the previous meal it may happen the alcohol is so active and powerful that it paralyzes the nerves of the heart and they call it heart failure.

Since unfired food is still live at the time it is eaten it is impossible for the yeast germ to invade it. Honey does not and can not ferment when combined with unfired food. Freshly flaked nuts do not ferment until four hours after they are immersed into liquid food and the juice of fresh fruit absorbs so readily that there is hardly a chance to ferment. Therefore those who live wholly on unfired food hardly know what indigestion means.

Now if the absence of fermentation means absence of indigestion, then it also means that unfired food is always digestible and easy of digestion ; because it is not known to ferment in the stomach when the stomach is clean and uncontaminated with cooked food.

There is only one chance for unfired fruit and nuts to ferment in the stomach and that is when the blood is withheld from the digestive circulation through fright, fear, anger, or any other exhaustive shock, and in such a case the toxins are so slight that it hardly ever produces a major disturbance. From experience it is found that alcohol produced from unfired fruits and nuts is less than one-tenth as toxic as that produced from any cooked food.

The greens are not known to ever have fermented in the stomach; and further than this, they are successfully used to clean out a sour stomach.

The unfired food re-encourages the functional nerves of digestion and finally promotes perfect assimilation.

The apyrtropher system does not advocate the eating of "RAW" foods, such as half-grown sour apples, quarter-grown tomatoes, unripe persimmons, dandelion roots or oysterplant-roots.

Try any of these and you will learn what "RAW" food is. The apyrtropher system also holds that all cooked food is irredeemably "raw" by being made fit for the "scavenger yeast germ" because the product of this germ paralyzes the functional nerves of digestion.

Dr. J Stevenson Hooker is right when he says (in the Food Reformers' Year Book for 1921, p. 28, second paragraph), "A very large percentage of people are wanting in perfect digestion, and these certainly could not do well on a raw dietary." He is right provided he corroborates the above meaning of "RAW," and if not, he has made an unwarranted statement for want of sufficient experience with the virtues of unfired food,"

IS COOKED FOOD NECESSAEY TO SUSTAIN A HIGH REASONING POWER?

Now since we have found that a higher reasoning power is the only difference between us and between our animal brothers and sisters, let us see whether a cooked diet is necessary to sustain or improve the reasoning power. When we feed our closest relatives, the monkeys, cooked food they get consumption, while when they are fed strictly on uncooked food they will reach their natural age in captivity. In the earlier part of this book I have given many other examples of different animals, who are not as closely related to us as the apes, who were suffering and an easier prey to disease when fed cooked food.

There is one great difference between the lower animals and us, the highest developed animals, which I did not mention before, and that is disease. We, with the greatest reasoning power, are constantly in need of professional advice and we are constantly suffering from disease, Year after year the colleges are "manufacturing"[11] more "'doctors", therefore it would be an injustice to say that we are solely suffering from disease, we are suffering equally as much from the people who live off of a sick suffering humanity.

There is a small percentage of us living on Unfired Food and this small percentage is never suffering from diseases or doctors, because they hardly ever become sick. It is unnecessary to mention that a well person has a superior reasoning power than a sick person. While all those who live on cooked (fired) food are always ailing. (Sick includes a little headache, a little cold, "all in", the dark-brown taste, the day after from the day before, nervous, and all the little pains here and there). I had to define the word "sick" because the average mortal is very modest when it comes to questions of health. This certain modesty is the only one which is universal among the members of the highest developed animate, the human beings. Disease is so common that the average person considers it a normal and necessary occurrence in human life. Everybody saves for a rainy day, which used to mean, when we get old, but we are more "civilized" now, and a rainy day now means when we get sick. The times when we used to get old are past, we are heroes now, we don't die like animals from old age. No! we die scientifically, on the operating table, if we have the money to pay for an operation. If we pull thru an operation, we can proudly show our friends our scars and let them praise our wonderful constitution and the skill of our butchers.

Today the poorest man can die scientifically; you don't have to die the old way, for there is a druggist on every corner who sells pills and dopes which are very beneficial to the owner of the store.

The idea of being sick is the most common and general topic of conversation besides the weather. The first thing the average person asks when he meets another, is: "How are you, your wife and family?", and if they are "all right", they answer with a sigh of relief, "glad to hear it."

We come to the conclusion now that cooked food and the prevalence of disease on one side, and uncooked food and the absence of disease on the other side, is the only real difference between the human animal with the highest reasoning power, and all the others with lower reasoning powers. Therefore I claim that cooked food is the cause of the majority of diseases, which I have shown in detail on pages 3 to 12 of this book.

HOW TO BEGIN THE UNFIRED DIET

The following utensils are necessary for the preparation of unfired food. Most of the utensils are in the average kitchen with a few exceptions. The utensils marked (*) are very useful but not essential for the beginner.

THE UTENSILS NECESSARY FOR PREPARING UNFIRED FOOD.

A chopping board 12x20 inches and

A cake knife with an 8-inch blade for chopping and mincing synede (salad) herbs.

- A shredder for cutting into neat and acceptable shreds, such as carrots, radishes, celeriac or parsley root, parsnip, sweet potato, kohl-rabi, cucumbers, apples and hard pears.
- A Drews "Flaker and Bromer" for flaking (grinding) combinations of dried fruits, cereal-meal and nuts for unfired bread and pie crusts and for flaking of nuts for salads. Do not try to grind hard cereals with the flaker, as it will break the shaft.
- A coarse grater for grating cocoanuts, horseradish, parsnips, cucumbers for soup and rhubarb stems for juice.
- A glass lemon juice burr.
- A 6-inch cake ring. "A Trophospeed" for quick grating and preparing unfired applesauce.
- A 3-inch cake ring.
- A rinsing pan for washing herbs and roots.
- An 8 or 9-inch pie plate, granite ware preferred.
- A 12-inch mixing bowl, granite ware preferred.
- A 4-pound scale, weighing in ounces.
- A table mill for grinding cereals and other dry material
- *A chopping bowl for chopping cabbage, cranberries and nuts and
- *A double bladed chopping knife.
- *An Enterprise Juice Extractor.

The utensils marked are not absolutely necessary and so it Is at your option to have them.

The flaker is the most important instrument for the preparation of unfired food. It is necessary for flaking nuts and the making of unfired bread and piecrust. There is no other machine which can be substituted for it, because this machine is especially designed for this purpose. Since these machines are guaranteed by the manufacturer, it does not pay to use a substitute.

You can extract juice by other methods, than by the use of the Enterprise Juice Extractor, but no other method is as economical and as speedy. The wonderful therapeutic value of vegetable and fruit juices is well known, but a Juice Extractor is necessary to extract, the juice from leaves, like spinach etc. Spinach juice with the addition of a little honey is a very wholesome tonic and food, for consumptives, and invalids.

Let us go to work now and prepare our first meal. We eat three meals per day, later you can suit yourself, the three meal plan I have found the most agreeable.

It is best to gradually begin with foods which are not commonly cooked, until you develop a taste for the more unusual foods. It is best to take a short fast of sixteen hours, before beginning the new diet.

The first recipe everyone will enjoy, it is a full satisfying meal as given here, the children will like, and prefer it over candy.

Take four ounces of seedless raisins and four ounces of almonds, or walnuts or unroasted peanuts, or take two medium size bananas mascerate them with a fork, add two ounces of flaked peanuts and a half teaspoonful of honey, mix well. Another good combination for beginners is a combination of Oatmeal with chopped peanuts and chipped dates.

Sliced Tomatoes with crushed nuts and dressed with honey.

Lettuce with chopped celery and fresh grated cocoanut

Shredded apple, mixed with seedless raisins and honey dressing.

For proportional combinations see the regular recipes in this book.

Before eating any of these meals read carefully the following article.

THE PSYCHOLOGY OF FEEDING!

When you are eating, you are feeding an individual. You must always bear this fact uppermost in your mind, while you are eating, and you will get better effects from the food you put into this individuals system.

Thoughts are live, real things so do not underestimate the power of thought. Regardless of how much you know about diet, how much information you get from this or any other work on diet, it will not do you the least bit of good unless you have the right mental attitude when you put the advice given into practice.

Let me demonstrate the power of thought in every day affairs, and you will be convinced that thoughts are material things in your life, with positive material effects.

You can not fill your stomach like the gas-tank of your flivver, because you are not a flivver, doing machine-work and going through the same operation all the time. You direct your actions by your mentality and the preciseness of these actions depends on the working condition of this mentality.

Your mentality is a powerful engine in the hands of an efficient operator, but if this powerful engine is left to itself it always plays havoc with the owner, and causes destruction to the property of the owner, i. e. your body, and if not restrained, in time will destroy itself and the owner will get insane or disintegrate.

It is your duty to constantly watch this powerful engine, your mind, so you are always conscious of the thoughts it is thinking. If it thinks thoughts harmful to the owner, it is the owners duty to stop this engine and correct the thoughts.

If the owner allows his mind to think harmful thoughts, these living thoughts will be put into actions, and actions can never be recalled, therefore hold the reigns of your thoughts tight, do not let your thoughts run at random.

Everything you create requires energy. Thoughts are creations of the mind. When your mind wanders, i. e. creates thoughts at random, you scatter your energy. Be careful not to scatter your energy, by consciously directing your thoughts and never allowing them to wander.

Become an expert operator of this wonderful engine, your mind; become a master of it, a Master-Mind.

Fear, doubt, hate, are all creations of the mind. They can not be seen, but they are as material as any matter you can see. They are real living things.

When you fear, when you doubt, when you hate, digestion is impaired. Because wrong thinking affects the circulation, and a wrong circulation immediately affects digestion, and the well-springs of life are poisoned.

Therefore it is self-evident to abstain from any food whatever, when you are in an agitated state of mind. You may have experienced the fact, that when you get excited, shocked, or worried you will lose your appetite. Be sure and heed nature's warning and abstain from food, when you are in such a condition.

When feeding your person always see that your mind is in a calm cheerful state. Always direct your thoughts to your activity. Do not eat and think about your work or read the newspaper. I know of an old lady, who can read, knit, talk and drink coffee at the same time. But she is really doing only one thing, i. e., knitting. She does not know what she reads, she talks nonsense, and she has to stop knitting when she drinks coffee, still she is very proud of her performance to be able to do four things at one time.

If you intend to become an old "Kaffee-schwester" (coffee sister), her course of action is advisable for you, but it is most everyone s desire to stay young as long as possible, and your age depends entirely on the state of your mind. At the moment you stop learning you begin to get old. You can only learn by concentration, by applying your mind to one thing at a time. If you do like this old lady, you scatter your mental energy. Whenever you scatter a force you weaken it. Can you now see how the average person weakens his mind?

Concentration of all energy results in more power, whether this is physical or mental energy. Can you now see how you can strengthen your mind?

When you feed your system and you consciously direct the food with your thoughts you will get greater benefit from this food, therefore be sure and re-enforce your food material with thought material from your brain. Enjoy every bite of your food, taste it, smell it and try to analyze every sensation you get from it. When eating unfired food for therapeutic purposes, concentrate on the effect it will have on your diseased condition while eating. This does not mean that Unfired food will not have its curative effect without direction of the mind, but by directing the mind you will get much quicker results and it is in your interest to get the quickest results possible.

Eat scientifically, do not fill your stomach like a potato sack, considering it full when it feels tight, and call this tightness satisfaction.

You can not insult your stomach that way, he will resent it and punish you when his opportunity arrives.

Those clean looking places with "four-legged chairs with one arm," where a person can wash down enough food in five minutes to create that customary tight feeling in the region of the waist, called satiated, are doing more financial good to the medical profession than anything I can think of. The Quick Lunchroom is a decided American institution and indigestion is a very decided American disease.

It is very common for a business man to wash or shove down his quick lunch in five minutes, so he can gain time enough to run over to the doctor's office to find out about his headache, pain in the stomach and gas which is troubling him so much, and have doc give him some pills or a prescription to stop that pain. Doc knows time is money, so he writes out a prescription in one minute and Mr. Businessman still has enough time in his lunch-hour to run over to the drug-store and have his prescription filled.

Poor, penny-wise business man! He saves minutes daily at his meals and these minutes cost him days, weeks or months in the hospital, on the operating table and often his life. It is true, time is money, for the "sanitary," germ-free-disease-producing Quick lunch room-owner, the doctor, the surgeon, the hospital arid the undertaker.

"Unfired food may be all right, but I am not sick," is a very common exclamation I hear, when I try to explain to a friend the benefits of natural living. This reminds me of a

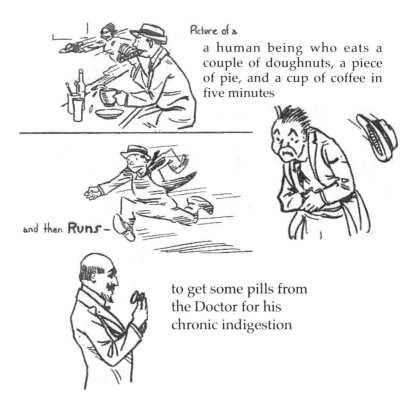

Picture of a human being who eats a couple of doughnuts, a piece of pie, and a cup of coffee in five minutes

and then Runs—

to get some pills from the Doctor for his chronic indigestion little vaudeville joke, which causes much laughter. A fool is asked by a man: "Hey, you want to make a Dime?" — "No Sir, I got Dime!

I should think that when a man gets advice how to keep well and he answers, "thank you, sir, but I am not sick" is more laughable than the vaudeville joke. But it has always been that way. People pay admission to enjoy some little jokers in vaudeville, but pass up... the biggest jokes in every day life. Very likely because they are usually comedians.

You do not have to wait until you are sick to derive some benefit from the Unfired Food; because the unfired diet has other advantages besides its curative value.

At present there is much complaint about the high cost of living. Wages are coming down, but very few of the necessities of life. There has been a reduction in Limousines, Seal Coats, Caviar, Silk Shirts and Silk Underwear. Five thousand Dollar furniture sets have been reduced to three-thousand dollars etc., but we common mortals do not get much benefit from such reductions.

The very same people who were not troubled on account of the high "war prices" are getting the greatest benefit from the postwar reduction Those who had their rent lowered, or their salary raised, need not read the following, until their rent is raised and their wages reduced.

If you live on Unfired Food, you need no heat for cooking and less heat to keep warm. In summer you need no fan to keep cool and you save electricity. You need no hot water and soap to wash your dishes and pans. If you put them in the sink and let the water run on them, they will be clean in a few minutes. You will save at least a quarter a week for cascarets, or pink pills, or you may have something better to force nature, if nature won't Pluto will, but in the long run Pluto won't and Nature won't, but the doctor and undertaker will. Nature always "will" when you live unfired, and it will everyday at the same hour and minute.

And all the time you save, it takes only a few minutes to prepare the unfired food, you can prepare a nice tasty dinner consisting of, soup vegetables, salad, pie, dessert etc., in 30 minutes. In five minutes you can prepare your breakfeast and eat it, you can have the same in the Quick-Lunch Room, but you get indigestion and constipation as a souvenir. You will miss these Souvenirs on the unfired diet.

I have lived the unfired way, and have found all these facts by experience, I have no desire to go back to the "old fashioned" way of living. After you live on the unfired diet for two months, I can assure you that you will never go back to cooked food, because you will have regained your natural taste. Cooked food is tasteless, and dead to the natural un-perverted taste.

There is one great mistake made, of which I must warn you dear reader. Many people made up their mind to try the unfired diet, but they did not get the least benefit from it; because they failed to study the principles of unfired feeding.

It takes a woman years of experimenting to learn how to cook, I do not ask the reader to spend years of practice to learn the preparation of unfired food, but it takes at least one week. If you begin the unfired diet with a potato, a carrot, a head of lettuce or a few onions, you will be disillusioned very soon and recommend Unfired Food to the cows, "but not for me."

Begin the diet gradually with things you commonly eat, bananas, tomatoes, lettuce, apples, berries etc.; but always be sure that you get 2 ozs. of nuts or almonds with each of your three daily meals. Some people complain that almonds are $1.00 per pound, use unroasted peanuts at 15c per lb., they will fit your pocketbook, better.

After you have tried the recipes given in this book, and have come to the conclusion that you will live the natural and only correct way, it will be advisable for you to get a copy of "Unfired Food & Trophotherapy," by Dr. Geo. J. Drews. This books contains over 300 recipes for the preparation of Unfired soups, drinks, vegetable salads, pies, bread, beer etc.

Your friends will be surprised when you offer them a piece of unfired pie, which is more delicious, than the best baked pie and can be made in ten minutes.

Anyone who contemplates to live the Unfired way should investigate carefully all the foregoing statements I have made in this book, for the purpose of contradicting them. When my statements are found correct, which they will be without question, the next step for the beginner will be to make up his or her mind to conscientiously live on the unfired diet for two months. After that time nothing in the world will induce them to return to the old mode of living except force.

There are many reasons given to the thinker for consideration, before starting the unfired diet. Those who take the Unfired diet for a fad of course do not need any reason. No more than they need a reason for wearing some unbecoming ridiculous style. Because someone they consider socially or otherwise important, does a thing, is enough reason for those "without reason."

PEPPERED FUN.

There is no difference between the beauty that eats "dead" food, and the maid that sweeps the dust under a beautiful carpet.

Not every girl can be a "Peach." You should worry, Beauty is only skin deep.

—But every girl can be clean.—

If you want cleanliness that is more than skin-deep, eat UNFIRED FOOD.

Worry is a hair remover, smoking a brain remover and Yeast, the latest mazuma remover.

The mothers who consider the sex-act filthy and immoral, should hide the evidence of such immoral acts and be ashamed of their babies.

RECIPES
HEALTH DRINKS.

The best and most natural health drink is pure crystalline water. Sometimes, however, it happens that the water may be contaminated with miasma and here is where lemon juice and other fruit juices and also rhubarb juice are of great value, as they are nature's sterilizers. The cocoanut milk is also a powerful sterilizer aside from its nutritiousness. Fruit juices are furthermore, useful in water for their relished flavors and for their harmless stimulant sugars. Drinks flavored or mixed with fresh herbal juices are called Saline Drinks. These drinks are of inestimable value to the sick and convalescent. They do not burden the stomach and yet furnish those purifying and tonic salts. When drinks contain some wholesome food element in dilute form they are called food drinks. These are often very useful No one should indulge in drinks right after a meal for they, then, dilute the gastric juices and disturb stomach digestion. Drinks at the temperature of the body and even a little warmer will prove to be most cooling in the end.

The best time to drink is three hours after a meal up to half an hour before the next meal There is an advantage in drinking thirty minutes before a meal, i. e., the liquid then entering the stomach becomes saturated with the gastric juices and then becomes an aid in the digestion of the following meal. Do not indulge in the drinks served at the soda fountain, for those drinks often, yes, too often, contain inorganic poisons for stimulation. Above all, beware of those drinks that are said to be refreshing. Yes, only refreshing. Ice cold drinks inflame the stomach and thereby cause an unnatural, unquenchable thirst. Tea, coffee, chocolate, beer and fresh milk are not wholesome drinks. The following recipes are intended to be served in an 8 oz. cup or glass. (From Unfired Food and Trophotherapy — Drews.)

LEMONADE

Put into a glass

$\frac{3}{4}$ oz. Lemon Juice (2 spoonful),

$\frac{1}{4}$ oz. Honey (teaspoonful) and fill up with Cold Water. Stir it well and serve.

ORANGEADE

Put into a glass

2 oz. Orange juice (14 cup),

$\frac{1}{2}$ oz. Honey (teaspoonful) and fill it up with Cold water. Stir it well and serve.

HERBADE

Soak in a cup of Water, for one or two hours

$\frac{1}{4}$ oz. Spearmint, mint, Fennel, Florence, Thyme, or Savory leaves. Use less if the dried herbs are fresh and strong. Strain the infusion and stir into it.

$\frac{1}{2}$ oz. Honey (teaspoonful) and serve.

Herbade promotes elimination through the kidneys. Cooked tea burdens the kidneys.

FRUIT FRAPPEE

With a table fork and in a shallow dish, macerate and beat to a creamy consistency

2 oz. Banana, Strawberries, large Plums or other soft fruit. Then put the beaten pulp into a cup, add

5 oz. Water and beat with a rotary beater until even. When the fruit is tart add

$\frac{1}{2}$ oz. Honey (teaspoonful) and serve.

Large quantities of fruit pulp may be made liquid by beating the pulp with the rotary beater after the fruit is macerated.

RHUBARBADE

3 oz. Rhubarb juice, extracted by grating the fresh stem, cut in two inch lengths.

$\frac{1}{4}$ oz. Honey (teaspoonful), beat into the juice, and add

$4\frac{1}{2}$ oz. Cold Water (or warm if desired).

TONIC DRINK

Mix

2 oz. Rhubarb juice (4 spoonful),

1 oz. Beet juice, extracted from grated beets or Swiss chard leafstalks,

$\frac{1}{2}$ oz. Honey (teaspoonful) and

$4\frac{1}{2}$ oz. Water, cold or warm, and serve.

For convalescents with a weak stomach I know no better remedy.

NEAR BUTTERMILK

Soak in a cup $\frac{3}{4}$ full of water

1 oz. Flax seed and beat it about every ten minutes during the course of one hour with a rotary eggbeater. Before beating the last time fill the cup nearly full with water and then let the seed settle. Meanwhile mix and rub into a cream

1 oz. Pignolias or Peanuts flaked exceedingly fine and

$\frac{1}{2}$ oz. Rhubarb Juice. Put this cream into a cup and add

$3\frac{1}{2}$ oz. Rhubarb Juice and beat it briskly with a rotary beater and then add

$3\frac{1}{2}$ oz. Flax seed fluid and beat it again briskly.

Now pour it through a large tea strainer, stirring a while, to keep it from clogging. Serve in a glass with a teaspoon or rye straw. At your option you may add a half ounce honey (teaspoonful).

"LEMONIZED" MILK

Into a cup containing
6 oz. Sweet milk pour
$\frac{3}{4}$ oz. Lemon juice (of half a lemon)

and quickly beat it briskly with a rotary eggbeater for two minutes to prevent it from curdling into lumps. This milk is acid sterilized. It is more wholesome for weaned children and adult convalescents than warm or sweet milk. Milk is not advised in the natural diet, but if it must be used let it be "lemon-ized" milk.

UNFIRED TONIC BEER

Mix together
3 oz. Powdered Sweetroot and
1 oz. Powdered Hop flowers.

Take a loose heaping teaspoonful of the mixture to a cup of water —stir—let it stand fifteen minutes or less—stir again—strain and serve. This unbrewed beer contains the full value of organic salts and organic sugar and so can in no wise be compared with the brewed and fermented or commercial beer.

$\frac{1}{2}$ oz. Powdered Sassafras bark may be added to the above to impart the flavor of root beer.

(For other recipes see Unfired Food and Tropho-therapy – Drews.)

COLD OR SUMMER SOUPS

PINEAPPLE SOUP

3 oz. Pineapple grated (i. e. pulp and juice) and
1 oz. Pignolias or Peanuts flaked.
Let it stand 15 min. and add
4 oz. Tomato minced or Cucumber grated and
$\frac{1}{2}$ oz. Olive Oil (spoonful) or Honey (teaspoonful.)
Beat well and serve.

CREAM OF TOMATO SOUP

Mix and beat together
- 6 oz. Tomato, peeled with a sharp knife, chipped and macerated with a fork,
- 1 oz. Peanuts or Pignolias flaked,
- $\frac{1}{2}$ oz. Parsley, Celery, Chives or other savory herbs minced and
- $\frac{1}{2}$ oz. Olive Oil (spoonful) and serve.

PANACEA SOUP.

Rub together
- 2 oz. Rhubarb—or Pineapple juice and
- 1 oz. Peanuts or Pignolias flaked, then add
- 2 oz. Cucumber peeled and grated,
- 2 oz. Tomato peeled and macerated with a fork,
- $\frac{1}{2}$ oz. Assorted Savory Herbs minced and
- $\frac{1}{2}$ oz. Olive Oil (spoonful) or Honey (teaspoonful).

Beat well and serve with an aluminum teaspoon.

SAVORY SOUP

Put into a soup bowl
- 7 oz. Tomato juice pulp,
- $\frac{1}{2}$ oz. Parsley or other savory herbs minced and
- $\frac{1}{2}$ oz. Olive Oil (spoonful). Beat the oil well into the stock and serve with an aluminum teaspoon.

CRANBERRY AND BEET OR PUMPKIN SOUP

Put into a soup bowl
- 1 oz. Cranberries chopped very fine and mashed with a wooden potato masher to free all the juice,
- 1 oz. Blood Beet, Pumpkin, Squash or Vegetable Marrow grated and
- 1 oz. Peanuts flaked or $\frac{1}{2}$ oz. Rolled Wheat. Rub these together and let it blend, then add

5 oz. Cucumber grated, Tomato macerated or in Winter Tepid Water and

$\frac{1}{2}$ oz. Honey (teaspoonful) or Olive Oil (spoonful). Beat well and serve.

BANANA SOUP

To

4 oz. Rhubarb juice add

$2\frac{1}{2}$ oz. Banana macerated to liquidity,

1 oz. Peanuts flaked and if desired

$\frac{1}{2}$ oz. Honey (teaspoonful). Stir to mix and serve.

WARM OR WINTER SOUPS

All the soups in which tepid water is used are intended for winter or whenever rhubarb, cucumbers or tomatoes can not be had. It is always best to let the water come to a boil and then allow to cool until it is below scalding temperature before it should be used. In order that the soup may not cool off too much in winter the soup bowl (consisting of heavy china), should be dipped into boiling water before the soup is filled into it. Heavy china holds the temperature better than thin porcelain

CRANBERRY SOUP

Take

2 oz. Cranberries, chop them fine in a chopping bowl, press all the juice out with a wooden potato masher and add

1 oz. Peanuts flaked or

$\frac{1}{2}$ oz. Oatmeal and $\frac{1}{2}$ oz. Parsley-root grated.

Rub all these together and let it stand 30 minutes. Then mix into it

4 oz. Tepid Water and

$\frac{1}{2}$ oz. Honey (teaspoonful) or Olive Oil (spoonful), beat well and serve.

CREAM OF CELERY SOUP.

Mix and mash together with a wooden potato masher
- 1 oz. Pecans or Peanuts flaked,
- $1\frac{1}{2}$ oz. Celery stalks or Cabbage chopped fine and
- $\frac{1}{2}$ Teaspoon Caraway seed ground and let it soak a while. Put this into a bowl and mix into it
- 5 oz. Tepid Water (not scalding hot) and, if desired
- $\frac{1}{2}$ oz. Honey (teaspoonful) or Olive Oil (spoonful) and serve.

BANANA CREAM SOUP.

Rub together
- $\frac{1}{2}$ oz. Lemon juice and
- 1 oz. Pignolias or Peanuts flaked. Let it blend a while and beat into it
- $1\frac{1}{2}$ oz. Banana macerated or Apple grated and
- $\frac{1}{2}$ Teaspoon Anise seed ground (optional)

Then add
- 5 oz. Tepid Water and as preferred
- $\frac{1}{2}$ oz. Honey (teaspoonful) or Olive Oil (spoonful).

Serve in a bouillon cup heated in boiling water.

CREAM OF PRUNE SOUP

Take
- 1 oz. Dried Prunes, mince and soak them 4 to 6 hours in
- 2 oz. Tepid Water. Then add to this
- 1 oz. Pignolias or Peanuts flaked
- $\frac{1}{2}$ Teaspoon Fennel or Anise seed ground (optional) and
- 4 oz. Tepid Water, not scalding. Beat and serve in a bowl heated in boiling water.

(For other recipes, see "Unfired Food and Trophotherapy" — Drews).

SALADS:

ASPARAGUS SALAD

APRIL

1 oz. Tender Asparagus tips sliced as fine as possible,
½ oz. Onion tips, chopped and
1 oz. Peanuts, Pignolias, Walnuts, Almonds
½ oz. Honey (teaspoonful) or Olive Oil (spoonful) and serve.

DANDELION SALAD

1½ oz. Dandelion leaves (and hearts) cut into shreds and chopped crosswise. Mix it with
1 oz. Cocoanut grated, Peanuts or Pignolias flaked or other nutmeats chopped and serve. When c hopped nuts are used.
½ oz. Olive Oil (spoonful or Honey (teaspoonful) may be added to advantage.

DANDELION SALAD

1½ oz. Dandelion leaves cut into shreds and chopped crosswise,
1 oz. Peanuts, Pignolias, Walnuts or Pecans chopped and
½ oz. Honey (teaspoon). Mix these well and to give it smoothness add
½ oz. Olive Oil (spoonful)

LENTILS IN NUT CREAM.

- 1 oz. Lentils soaked over night, rinsed, and dried in a towel,
- ½ oz. Pignolias or Peanuts flaked and
- 2 oz. Rhubarb juice. Mix these and beat it to a creamy consistency and serve with an aluminum teaspoon. For variety add
- ½ oz. Honey (teaspoonful) just before serving.

ASPARAGUS IN NUT CREAM.

- 1½ oz. Asparagus tips, cut as thin as a knife blade. Use tender tips only.
- 1 oz. Pignolias or Peanuts, flaked,
- 1 oz. Rhubarb juice. Mix these and beat until creamy. Just before serving add
- ½ oz. Honey (teaspoonful); mix again and serve.

Serve without honey if preferred or replace it with Olive Oil.

ARTICHOKE SALAD

- 1½ oz. Artichokes, washed, cubed or chopped,
- ½ oz. Onion minced and
- 1 oz. Pignolias flaked or chopped or cocoanut grated. Mix these well and serve.

DANDELION FLOWER SALAD
(A Good Tonic)

- 2 oz. Dandelion Flowers cut fine. Lay a bunch of flowers on the board and cut thin slices from the bunch cutting each flower through several times. Use the stems also.
- 1 oz. Cocoanut grated, Pignolias or Peanuts flaked.

Toss these well together and serve garnished with a flower or two. This is a delicious dish. Dandelions blossom a second time in September and October.

MAY
LETTUCE AND COCOANUT SALAD.

Mix

$2\frac{1}{2}$ oz. Lettuce cut into shreds and these cut again with

1 oz. Cocoanut grated and drip over it

2 oz. Cocoanut Milk. Serve with a teaspoon.

SPINACH AND COCOANUT SALAD

Mix

$2\frac{1}{2}$ oz. Spinach cut into shreds and these cut again with

1 oz. Cocoanut grated and drip over it

2 oz. Cocoanut Milk. Serve with a teaspoon.

COMBINATION SALAD

2 oz. Lettuce cut into shreds and then chopped crosswise,

$\frac{1}{4}$ oz. Onion Tips cut fine,

$\frac{1}{2}$ oz. Curled Garden Cress cut fine and

1 oz. Flaked Peanuts. Toss and mix the nuts well into the salad and pour over it,

2 oz. Rhubarb juice. Serve it thus or beat it till the nuts become creamy.

RADISH SALAD

Mix

$\frac{1}{2}$ oz. Radishes cubed or chopped with

$\frac{1}{2}$ oz. Peanuts, Pignolias or other nuts chopped or flaked. For black or other very hot radishes use one whole ounce of nuts. Garnish with a few thin slices.

LINDEN SALAD.

1 oz. **Young Linden Leaves** cut into shreds and minced and

1 oz. **Peanuts** (or other nuts) flaked. Toss these together and serve.

YARROW IN NUT CREAM.

1 oz. **Young Yarrow leaves**, cut on a chopping board as fine as possible,

1 oz. **Peanuts** flaked, and

2 oz. **Rhubarb juice**. Beat these until it is creamy, then add and mix into it

$\frac{1}{2}$ oz. **Honey** (teaspoonful) and

$\frac{1}{2}$ oz. **Olive Oil** (spoonful). Serve only on request and with an aluminum teaspoon.

PLANTAIN SALAD

$1\frac{1}{2}$ oz. Plantain cut into shreds and minced and

1 oz. Peanuts or Pignolias flaked. Mix and serve— or, with your favorite nuts chopped, you may add

$\frac{1}{2}$ oz. Honey (teaspoonful).

JUNE
LETTUCE AND CRESS SALAD

2 oz. Lettuce cut into shreds and chopped

1 oz. Curled Garden Cress chopped fine and

1 oz. Cocoanut grated, Pignolias or Peanuts flaked. Mix these garnish and serve.

LETTUCE AND PARSLEY SALAD.

$1\frac{1}{2}$ oz. Lettuce, cut into shreds and cut again and

1 oz. Parsley cut and minced. Toss these together and serve with

1 oz. Honey (2 teaspoonful).

KOHL-RABI SALAD

- $1\frac{1}{2}$ oz. **Kohl-rabi** diced or chopped,
- $\frac{1}{2}$ oz. **Onion Tips**.
- 1 oz. **Cocoanut** grated, Peanuts or Pignolias flaked or other nutmeats chopped. Toss these into one another and serve with the chopped nuts.
- $\frac{1}{2}$ oz. **Olive Oil** (spoonful) or Honey (teaspoonful) may be used.

RADISH AND BEAN SALAD.

- 1 oz. **Kohl-rabi** and
- 1 oz. **String-beans** sliced as thin as possible and
- 1 oz. **Peanuts**, Pignolias or Almonds flaked or Cocoanut grated. Toss these together and serve.

GREEN PEAS IN NUT CREAM

- $1\frac{1}{2}$ oz. **Tender Peas**, whole
- $\frac{1}{2}$ oz. **Savory herbs**, minced
- 1 oz. **Peanuts** (or other nuts) flaked and
- 2 oz. **Rhubarb juice**, extracted by grating the fresh stems cut in 2 in. lengths. Mix and beat these to the proper consistency and serve with an aluminum teaspoon.

JULY SALAD

- 1 oz. **Young Sweet Corn**, sliced, off the cob,
- 1 oz. **Endive**,
- 1 oz. **Peanuts** or Mixed Nuts chopped. Mix into these
- $\frac{1}{2}$ oz. **Olive Oil** (spoonful) or Honey (teaspoonful) and chip it over it
- 2 oz. **Tomatoes**.

STUFFED CANTALOUPE

Fill the natural cavity of a

- 5 oz. **Half Cantaloupe** with the following mixture
- $\frac{1}{2}$ oz. **Parsley**, Celery or Oxalis, minced and
- 1 oz. **Pignolias** or Peanuts flaked.

SPINACH-BEET SALAD

- $\frac{1}{2}$ oz. **Spinach-beet leaves** cut into shreds and chopped,
- $\frac{1}{4}$ oz. **Savory herbs** minced or Onion chopped and
- $\frac{1}{2}$ oz. **Peanuts** chopped. Mix these well with
- $\frac{1}{4}$ oz. **Olive Oil** (teaspoonful) and serve.

At another dinner when serving the same dish add and mix into it

- $\frac{1}{2}$ oz. **Honey** (teaspoonful.)

MOCK SAUERKRAUT

- 3 oz. **Crisp Cabbage** shredded and chopped
- $\frac{1}{2}$ Teaspoon **Caraway** seed ground,
- 2 oz. **Rhubarb juice**, extracted by grating the fresh stems cut in 2 inch lengths,
- $\frac{1}{2}$ oz. **Honey** (teaspoonful). Mix the liquid well into the slaw and serve.

WATERMELON

Serve a

- 2 lb. **Watermelon** section in a plate with a knife and fork.

AUGUST
TOMATO AND CUCUMBER SANDWICHED SALAD
3 oz. **Cucumber**, peeled and sliced,
3 oz. **Tomato** sliced and
1 oz. **Nutmeats** flaked.

Put a layer of flaked nutmeats on each slice of cucumber and cover them with a slice of tomato. Arrange the sandwiches artistically on lettuce, endive or parsley and serve.

STUFFED TOMATO
Cut a

6 or 8 oz. **Tomato** in two then cut out part of the central pith and serve it for capping. Now scrape out the partition walls, seeds and juice and mix this with

1 oz. **Peanuts** or Pignolias flaked and
$\frac{1}{2}$ oz. **Celery** or Parsley minced. Refill the halves with this mixture, cover with the piths reversed and serve.

SWEET CORN SALAD
$2\frac{1}{2}$ oz. **Green Sweet Corn** sliced off the cob with a sharp knife and the remaining pulp scraped out with the back of the knife and

1 oz. **Pignolias** or Peanuts flaked, Cocoanuts grated or other nuts chopped.

Mix these and serve on an endive or lettuce leaf.

PIGNOLIAS POTATO SALAD
2 oz. **Potatoes**, peeled, sliced and chopped
1 oz. **Pignolias** flaked, mix and spread on a lettuce leaf then sprinkle over it
1 oz. **Rhubarb juice** and serve.

This dish will relieve and cure Kidney troubles when all cooked starches are avoided.

VARIETY SALAD

- ½ oz. Bean-pods or Young Peas,
- ½ oz. Potato
- ½ oz. Carrot or Beet,
- ½ oz. Onion or Celery all chopped to the size of corn and
- 1 oz. Pignolias or Peanuts flaked or other Nut-meats chopped. Toss all together and serve with the chopped nuts
- ½ oz. Olive Oil (spoonful) may be added.

GREEN TOMATO AND CRESS SALAD

- 2 oz. Green Tomato chipped,
- 1 oz. Upland or Water Cress or Nasturtium Leaves cut into shreds and minced and
- 1 oz. Peanuts or Pignolias flaked or chopped. Toss these together and serve or when the nuts are chopped
- ½ oz. Olive Oil (spoonful) or Honey (teaspoonful) may be added.

SQUASH SALAD

- 3 oz. Summer Squash or Vegetable Marrow cut into dice and
- 1 oz. Pignolias, Almonds or Peanuts flaked. Mix these and serve or improve it by dripping over it
- 2 oz. Rhubarb juice (4 spoonfuls.)

TOMATO SUPAWN

- 2 oz. Tomato chipped
- ½ oz. Carrot or Sweet Potato grated
- ½ oz. Black Walnuts or other nut meats chopped
- ½ oz. Parsley minced and
- 1 oz. Young Sweet Corn sliced off the cob or Young Peas chopped. Stir these to a pudding and serve.

ICE-PLANT SALAD

Mix

- 3 or 4 oz. Ice-plant, chopped with
- 1 oz. Peanuts or Pignolias flaked and rub or macerate enough to moisten the nuts, and then add
- $\frac{1}{2}$ oz. Honey (teaspoonful).

SEPTEMBER
LIMA BEAN AND PUMPKIN SALAD

- 1 oz. Young Lima Beans chopped
- 1 oz. Squash or Pumpkin chopped or cubed
- $\frac{1}{2}$ oz. Onion, Parsley or Sweet Pepper chopped and
- 1 oz. Peanuts or Pignolias flaked.

Toss these together and serve.

VEGE-FRUIT SALAD

Cut small Cantaloupes or Muskmelons in halves, scrape out the pulp leaving the rind whole and refill with the following mixture:

- 2 oz. Muskmelon or Cantaloupe pulp,
- 1 oz. Tomato minced and
- 1 oz. Nut Meats flaked. Serve with a teaspoon.

SELECTED SALAD

- 1 oz. Endive cut into shreds and chopped crosswise,
- 1 oz. Cabbage shredded and chopped and
- $\frac{1}{2}$ oz. Peanuts flaked. Mix these and chip over it
- 2 oz. Cucumber and add
- $\frac{1}{2}$ oz. Honey (teaspoonful). Now toss it all to mix and serve.

NUT CREAM SLAW

1 oz. Potato, peeled, sliced, 1 oz. Cabbage, shredded,
$\frac{1}{2}$ oz. Onion, sliced. Put all these in a chopping bowl and chop till fine, then add
1 oz. Peanuts or other nuts flaked.
$\frac{1}{2}$ Teaspoonful caraway seed and
2 oz. Rhubarb juice or cucumber juice, produced by putting through juice extractor.

Mix and beat all together to a creamy consistency and serve. Any two vegetables on hand may be used to make this slaw.

OCTOBER SALAD

$\frac{1}{2}$ oz. Cabbage cut into shreds and chopped,
$\frac{1}{2}$ oz. Potato chopped
$\frac{1}{2}$ oz. Celery, Parsley, Onion, Oxalis or Sorrel minced
2 oz. Tomato chipped and
1 oz. Nut Meats chopped
$\frac{1}{2}$ oz. Honey (teaspoonful) or Olive Oil (spoonful). Mix well and serve.

FALL SALAD

This salad comes in handy when the lettuce season is over.

1 oz. Parsnip or Parsley Root grated,
1 oz. Peanuts flaked and
1 oz. Endive (smooth or curled), Scorzonera leaves Parsley, Celery (leaves and stalks), Chicory leaves, Dandelion, Nasturtium leaves or Upland Cress cut into shreds and minced. Mix the three and drip over it
$\frac{1}{2}$ oz. Olive Oil (spoonful), mix again, garnish and serve.

ARTICHOKE AND SWEET PEPPER SALAD

$1\frac{1}{2}$ oz. Artichokes diced or chopped,
1 oz. Sweet Salad Pepper or Tomato chipped,
1 oz. Peanuts or Pignolias flaked or other nut meats chopped and if on hand
$\frac{1}{4}$ oz. Parsley, Leek or Celery minced. Toss these together and serve.

KALE SALAD

1 oz. Curled Kale or Chinese Cabbage chopped and
1 oz. Peanuts, Pignolias or Almonds flaked.
Mix these and serve.
Learn to like this salad for the sake of your blood.

SELECTED SALAD

1 oz. Egg-plant chipped,
1 oz. Sweet Pepper chipped or Celery chopped or minced,
1 oz. Young Lima Beans, chopped,
$\frac{1}{2}$ oz. Olive Oil (spoonful) and
$\frac{1}{2}$ oz. Honey (teaspoonful) Mix the dressing well into the salad and serve.

CABBAGE AND BANANA SALAD

2 oz. Cabbage cut into shreds and chopped,
1 oz. Celery stalks chopped and
2 oz. Banana chipped. Stir these until the banana becomes nearly fluid and serve.

CAULIFLOWER AND CHICK PEA SALAD

- 1 oz. Cauliflower tops or Cabbage chopped
- 1 oz. Chick Peas or Green Peas soaked till soft and chopped
- $\frac{1}{4}$ oz. Celery or Parsley minced (if on hand)
- $\frac{1}{2}$ oz. Honey (teaspoonful) or Olive Oil (spoonful)
- ($\frac{1}{4}$ oz. Oil added to the honey may please some palates exceedingly.)

Mix the honey or oil well into the salad and serve.

PEA AND CABBAGE SALAD

- 1 oz. Soaked Green Peas chopped
- $1\frac{1}{2}$ oz. Cabbage cut into shreds and chopped and
- 1 oz. Pignolias flaked or other nut meats chopped. Mix these and serve, with chopped nuts
- $\frac{1}{2}$ oz. Honey (teaspoonful) or Olive Oil (spoonful) may be added to advantage.

LENTILS IN HONEY

- 1 oz. Lentils, soaked overnight, rinsed and dried in a towel and
- $\frac{1}{2}$ oz. Honey (teaspoonful). Mix the honey into the lentils and serve immediately.

LIMA BEANS IN WINTER

Soak lima beans until soft and then slip them out their coats. Chop

- 1 oz. Blanched Beans and mix them with
- 1 oz. Cocoanut grated or Pignolias or Almonds flaked; This dish is wholesome but still better when
- 1 oz. Chopped Celery, or Cabbage is added.

SIMPLICITY SALADS

Pile neatly into a proper dish

- 4 oz. Washed Lettuce and set beside it a small dish with
- 1 oz. Pignolias or other shelled nuts. Mix the juices of both while chewing.
- 2 oz. Radishes (five small red radishes) laid on a lettuce leaf covered with
- 1 oz. Whole Peanuts or other shelled nuts and serve with a teaspoon. When the ensalivated nut juice is chewed into the radish juice the hottest radish will not bite.
- 3 or 4 oz. Dates, Figs, Raisins, Pears or Prunes with an addition of
- 1 oz. Peanuts or other nutmeats. Mix the juice of the nuts and fruit while chewing and enjoy the blended flavors.

BANANA RELISH

Drip over

- 3 oz. Banana chips mixed with
- 1 oz. Nuts, chopped
- $\frac{1}{4}$ oz. Lemon juice (teaspoonful) and serve.

WINTER FRUIT SAUCE

After washing the proper quantity of Dates, Figs, Prunes, Pears, Raisins or Currants take

- 2 oz. Dried Fruit, mince it and soak it in
- $2\frac{1}{2}$ oz. Water over night or till soft and then add
- $\frac{1}{2}$ oz. Nutmeats chopped or Cocoanut grated. Mix and serve.

WINTER FRUIT SALAD

Mix

- 2 oz. Apple, Banana or Orange chipped with
- 1 oz. Raisins or chipped Figs or Dates and
- 1 oz. Pignolias flaked or other Nutmeats chopped and serve.

MINCE-FRUIT

Put into a chopping bowl

- $1\frac{1}{2}$ oz. Seeded or Seedless Raisins, (6) Dates, Figs or Dried Pears and
- 1 oz. Walnuts, Pignolias, Pecans, Almonds, Brazil Nuts, Filberts, Chestnuts, Peanuts or Mixed Nutmeats and chop until there is nothing larger than a lentil. Serve this plain, with fresh fruit or mixed with meal.

UNFIRED POUNDCAKE

- 20 oz. Sweet Corn, Wheat, Hulless Barley, Rice Corn or Rice ground to meal and
- 12 oz. Dates or Figs chopped in part of the above meal. Mix all the meal and chopped fruit and run it through the flaker twice. The second time do not let the flakes pile up and become a mass. Mix and work into the flakes
- 4 oz. Prunes or dark Raisins chopped and
- 4 oz. Almonds or Peanuts chopped. Now press and pound this mass hard into a 6 inch cake ring or four 3 inch muffin rings lined with paper. Set it aside to harden and slice with a sharp knife in a sawing motion. This cake improves by age.

(For other recipes see Unfired Food & Tropho-therapy Drews).

PIE FILLINGS

The weights of the ingredients of the following pie fillings are so computed that the final combination will just fill a common nine inch pie plate. If more than one pie is to be made the weight of each ingredient is to be multiplied by the number of pies intended. These recipes have been tested for exactness and good results.

APPLE CREAM PIE

Crust 8 oz.

6 oz. Sweet Corn Meal and

3 oz. Currants. Mix and run through the flaker. Spread the resulting dough into a slightly oiled plate. Filling 16 oz.

7 oz. Apple, grated and

$3\frac{1}{2}$ oz. Pignolias, flaked. Mix and beat these into a cream, add

6 oz. Apple, cubed, mix again and spread over the above crust. Garnish with four or six ornamental apple slices and cut into 4 or 6 sections. One quarter of this pie equals a full and wholesome meal.

PRUNE OR PLUM PIE

Crust 8 oz. Filling 16 oz.

5 oz. Pignolias or peanuts flaked and

11 oz. Fresh Prunes or plums chipped off the stone with a sharp knife.

Mix and rub these to a creamy consistency leaving as much of the chips unmashed as possible and fill into crust.

APPLE AND BANANA PIE

Crust 8 oz. Filling 16 oz.

7 oz. Apple, grated and

$3\frac{1}{2}$ oz. PIgnolias, flaked. Mix and beat these into a cream, add

6 oz. Banana, cubed, mix again and spread into the crust. Cut into four or six sections and serve.

(For other recipes see Unfired Food & Tropho-therapy — Drews.)

BANANA MOUSSE

Macerate with a silver fork until liquid

2 oz. Banana and then stir into it

1 oz. Strawberries quartered or bruised, small tomato chips, orange chipped or small raisins and serve.

MIXED FRUIT SAUCE

Stir together

1 oz. Oranges chipped,

1 oz. Peaches chipped,

1 oz. Plums chipped,

$\frac{1}{4}$ oz. Pignolias flaked and

$\frac{1}{2}$ oz. Honey (teaspoonful) and serve.

This dish can be composed of other fruits in their season.

(For other recipes see Unfired Food & Trophotherapy — Drews.

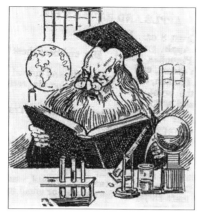

Are you awake? Consider me an authority, ossified, whiskered, with high self-esteem who thinks "I am always right and I can force my opinion on you, because I know you dare not challenge me."

CREPE HANGERS HYMN.
"I have a lot of trouble,
But I wouldn't be without it;
I find it such a comfort
To tell other folks about it."

If I woke you up, you will challenge every statement I make and try to refute it; if you cannot refute it, you can give me credit; but do not think, because I have been right this time, that I am unable to make a mistake the next time. Keep on fighting and you will protect yourself from illusions, and you will do me a great favor by protecting me from self-esteem and ossification.

MEAT

The fatal belief that meat is a necessary article of diet and that the animal world has been created for the purpose of furnishing man with food is one of the many superstitions which have been handed down to us from generation to generation.

The nourishing constituents of meat—fat and protein—are contained in much better and purer condition and in more equal proportions in the various products of the soil, furnishing us with all that is necessary to keep us in perfect health, as long as we enjoy them in their natural "unfired" state.

Nuts and certain legumes, the peanut for instance, are more nutritious than the best meat, they are much cheaper, and they contain no impurities which have to be eliminated by the kidneys and the other depurative organs.

Meat is decayed animal matter. The process of decomposition (decay) begins soon after the animal is dead. By putting the cadaver of a pig ox or lamb on ice does not stop the process of decaying, it only retards it. This fact is well known to the butchers, and accounts for some of the different qualities of meat. First class meat which is usually bright red (very little decayed), costs quite a little more than the dark red and often black meat sold in the congested quarters of the large cities where the poorer classes exist. In summertime these cheaper grades of meat emanate an unmistakable odor of decay.

It may be disgusting to some of the readers to be reminded of facts and conditions like the above, but it ought not be as disagreeable to read these facts than to make meals of decayed animal cadavers every day.

The meat as used in the "reasonable" priced restaurants are usually of the "dark red" and "black" quality, such as pork chop sandwiches sold at ten cents, Hamburger sandwiches at fifteen cents, etc.

Of course there are many people who are not very particular what they eat. But I am not writing this for the people who do not care how things look before they reach the table, "as long as they taste good."

Often when I tell people about the filthy past of an appetizing (?) steak, they plug their ears with their fingers and say: "I don't care what happens behind the kitchen-door, please keep still; you spoil my appetite." They always remind me of the ostrich who hides his head in the sand.

Regardless how little the "damphool" in your upper story knows about the true conditions of the food you eat, you can fool "him" upstairs, but not the chemist—your stomach.—Your stomach lacks imagination, it has no eyes nor taste, it has only one sense, i. e. that of analyzing foods, and this sense never fails. Stop trying to fool your stomach.

"If you do hard work you have to eat meat' is a common expression. Let us see whether such is true. The average person considers manual work like shoveling coal, farm work, sawing wood etc., hard work; brain work, office work, needle work etc., light occupation. Space does not permit to discuss the falsity of this conception.

Prof. Voit of Munich has found, by careful investigations, carried on for a number of years, that: heat and energy are almost exclusively created by carbohydrates and fats. We do not eat meat for carbohydrates, but for the protein contained in it. Meat does not contain any carbohydrates. Professor Voit found further, that even at the most strenuous work the body consumes no more protein than when at rest and that the average man can get along fairly well on about one ounce of protein per day.

Let us not take a man's word for anything because he is a professor. Let us see whether we can not prove the fact that meat is unnecessary in the performance of what is commonly accepted as hard work.

The Chinese Kuli is preferred by any captain, over the white worker when it comes to hard work. For instance, the loading or unloading of cargoes. The Kuli works 14 hours and often up to 20 hours; he never partakes of meat; and his food consists of rice and fruit.

In spite of the hard work, and the frugal meals, disease is practically an unknown quantity among the kulis.

I have shown that man is able to do hard work without meat-eating, but I will show you now the injurious effects of meat in a similar manner.

The diet of the inhabitants of Iceland, in the northern Atlantic ocean, consists almost exclusively of animal food of which fish, either fresh or dried, form by far the largest proportion. During the summer they have butter and milk in considerable abundance; but of bread, fruit or any other vegetable food there is the utmost scarcity, and among the lower classes an almost entire privation. As an effect of these circumstances in the mode of life of the Icelanders, skin diseases arising from improper nutrition, are very frequent among them, and appear under some of their worst forms. Scurvy and leprosy are common in the Island, occurring especially on the western coast where the inhabitants depend chiefly upon fishing, and where the pastures are inferior in extent and produce. Inflammatory affections of the abdominal viscera and disposition to worms are likewise very common among the Icelanders, in consequence of the peculiar diet to which they are accustomed.

If we need only one ounce of protein per day, what becomes of the large quantities of protein partaken of by the average person in the form of eggs, meat, etc., per day? That "excessive amount of protein causes a large number of diseases," is a well known fact.

A pound of meat consists of three-fourths of impure water, and this impure water has to be eliminated by the depurative organs, liver, kidneys, skin, etc., leaving only four ounces of water for food. Then too, meat aside from the fact that it is unwholesome is one of the most expensive foods.

When we compare a pound of unroasted peanuts at 45 cents to a pound of meat costing about the same, we find that the nuts contain on an average 90 per cent of nourishment and no waste matter which has to be eliminated, while meat contains only 20 per cent of nourishment, and much waste matter.

I have shown that meat is not necessary for the well being of the individual. I have also shown that nuts replace meat in a superior fashion; because they are not saturated with the waste products of muscle and nerve, which intoxicate delicate persons, like alcohol. The average person does not consider that meat contains uric acid, (Urine).

You need about one (1) ounce of protein or albumen per day, there is no good reason why you should indulge in the customary large quantities of food containing this product. You get many times that quantity of protein or albumen, causing you great suffering, through albumen poisoning.

Protein waste, or albumen poisoning, manifests itself through rheumatism, ptomaine poisons, varied conditions of autointoxication, etc.

If you wish to build an ideal home for scavengers, eat plenty of meat and eggs. Decomposed proteids (meat and eggs) are wonderful "germ-food," and if you want disease-germs to be healthy and thrive it is of utmost importance to make a "garbage-container" out of your stomach and intestines, but, if you eat only pure, natural (unfired) food the poor germs will starve to death.

People are getting more and more educated to the fact that meat is harmful and the consumption of meat is getting lower every year. This is a well known fact and the packing concerns are making strenuous propaganda through the press and posters, to counteract this. It is nothing unusual to find a large "paid" ad telling the public about the value of meat eating, and in a little obscure corner of the same issue an article from an authority discouraging the use of meat.

"The doctor told me I should not eat any meat," said a lady of my acquaintance, "so I eat only chicken." Chicken is not considered meat, by many people, who try to fool their doctor. Most of them know very well that there is no difference, but they are "wise fools."

If you are in doubt whether fish is in the same class as meat, because it is "so" clean, living in water, just go within ten feet of dead fish at your beach or river, which has been exposed to the beneficial rays of the sun for a few hours, and you will find that you are not very enthusiastic about the fresh "sea-breeze."

If you eat meat and your digestion is impaired, your stomach may not be burdened for all the poisonous matter out of the "scavenger food," and some of the poison may leave your system without harming you. In order to avoid this, by all means eat soup. Soup will give you every drop of "urine" in the meat, nothing will go to waste. If meat will not kill you, eat meat soup three times a day, seven times per week, it will do the work.

Some time ago I read a book by a well known doctor who disapproves of meat eating in general; but his assistants eat meat. He claims in giving treatments to the sick "animal-magnetism" is necessary, and that his operators get this necessary element through meat-eating.

I consider magnetism a form of life, but this doctor is a wonder, he gets magnetism from the flesh of dead animals. (A new variety of "scientific" nonsense, sprung on the unsuspecting public.)

Is it not a grand and glorious feeling, to know that your stomach is the graveyard for dead animals, and the hunting-ground of the "intestinal hyena," the disease-germ?

CEREALS

You can live on whole wheat and water entirely; but whole wheat and all other cereals are hard to digest. Cereals are not advisable for people with a weak stomach, and even after your stomach becomes normal through the use of un-fired food they are unnecessary, because we have so many other foods to take the place of cereals which are easier digested.

There are a few recipes given where whole wheat flour is used, in the unfired bread for instance. If you eat whole cereals they have to be masticated very thoroughly, and it is necessary for you to be out in the open air and to have plenty of exercise, or hard work.

Never soak wheat or other cereals; because they ferment very easily in the warm stomach, they act similar as the soaked cereals which are used for making whiskey.

BREAD

You will find on many bakers windows: "Bread is your best food, eat more of it." This is another one of many lies to commercialize a harmful product.

Beware of white bread; it is not pure food but very "poor" food. White bread in the following combinations is the cause of a great deal of indigestion: Hot rolls, coffee and rolls, "fresh bread hot from the oven," etc. Beware of it.

One of the latest disease producers and a good money producer for the manufacturer is yeast. Yeast causes dyspepsia! It has no beneficial action for the person who takes it. Do not be misled by billboards and advertising signs telling you different, as these advertisements are paid for by the Yeast manufacturer.—Think!

SUGAR A DISEASE PRODUCER

The free use of unnatural sugar, i. e. refined white cane sugar, candy, molasses, brown sugar, etc., by children, lays the foundation of lifelong ills. This is true when the sugar is pure, not mentioning the grossly adulterated sugar in cheap candy.

Candy stores are opening daily and they are all doing a tremendous business. Candy eating has become a habit, and the man or woman that eats candy, is harmed more, and should be considered a greater fiend than the tobacco fiend; because tobacco is less poisonous and the consequences are not as disastrous as those from sugar-eating. (I do not smoke, and do not approve of smoking).

The cause of the great consumption of sugar in form of candy pastries etc., is malnutrition, starvation of the cells and nerves; the starved system cries for food to replace the nervous and physical wear and tear, and the ignorant fool in the upper story, feeds the starving system poison in form of sweets.

Sugar is responsible for more physical ills than alcohol. Go into the candy kitchen and you will find copper utensils. Why? Because sugar attacks and destroys iron. What will the sugar do to the iron in your blood? Notice the pale anemic office worker, who sends the "kid" every afternoon for a bag of candy, and whose lunch consists of an ice cream soda or sundae, a white bread sandwich and a piece of pie and sweetened coffee.

Sugar is a strong irritant. As soon as you take the least amount of it into your mouth you cause a catarrh, (slime); if you want to prove this to yourself put some into your nostrils. Can you see the cause of inflammation of the tonsils? Most people suffering from growth in the nose (adenoids) are heavy sugar eaters.

A prohibition of the sale of candies would put fifty percent of all the dentists out of business within three years. Surgery would become less profitable and indigestion less common.

The Hootch-maker adds sugar to get more alcohol from his mash. You add sugar to the "mash" in your stomach and you will get the same effect. Sugar taken in large quantities will not be absorbed by the system and whatever stays in the system unabsorbed, will be absorbed by the yeast germ. If your system becomes a "yeast-germ-incubator," it ceases to be a "Home of Health."

Give refined sugar to a native and he will spit it out with disgust, the taste for refined sugar has to be acquired the same as the taste for tobacco.

The cook can not get along without sugar; but the "Apyrtropher" (unfired fooder) uses honey instead. Honey has all the sweetening properties of sugar without its faults. At present Honey is the only NATURAL sugar, I know of.

In the average household honey is classed with castor oil, liniment and peroxide. This is a great injustice to the bee; because honey is not a drug. It is not poisonous like castor oil, or useless like liniment or peroxide. Give the little ones plenty of honey it will not harm them; but beware of "wholesome candy."

When you meet a person that always brags about his honesty, truth and kindness, you get suspicious, so do the same when you read the words "wholesome," "home made" etc., on articles of food. Look into the matter.

Fruits contain a great deal of wholesome sugar (grape sugar) and if the children crave for sweets give them some dried dates, figs, prunes or raisins. The yet un-perverted taste of the child will always prefer these natural sweets over candy.

Many parents, who understand the harmful effect of sugar, have the mistaken idea that plain chocolate or milk chocolate, are wholesome sweets. Chocolate contains two harmful, substances instead of one, i. e. sugar and cocoa.

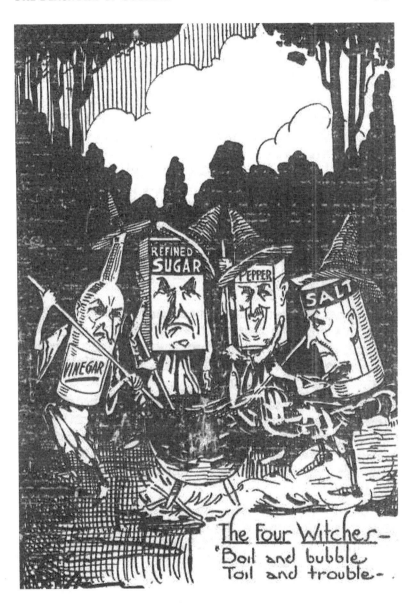

The Four Witches—
"Boil and bubble,
Toil and trouble—."

    Men who work in the big sugar refineries are notoriously short-lived. THINK!!
    Fruit-sugar, honey, (natural sweets) can safely be eaten by people suffering from diabetes. Beware of saccharine.

SALT

In our "enlightened" age we smile at the superstitions of our ancestors. Many years hence we shall be the laughing stock of the future generations because we believed that salt, (the inorganic mineral, chloride of sodium) is a necessary addition to our daily food.

Salt eating, is a habit, just like the tobacco, alcohol, coffee, or dope habit; or the latest "yeast eating" habit.

Salt is as wholesome and necessary as meat. It is the ally of meat in the destruction of health. Salt hides the insipidness of meat. Add some salt to dead, decayed animal matter, (meats, sausages etc.) and it becomes wholesome (?) food.

Salt is the same to the butcher and cook, as rouge is to the savage female, or a high collar to the dirty-necked male; it covers filthy, unsanitary, disagreeable conditions; which could otherwise be detected by the un-perverted natural taste. It is the magic wall of the cook; it conceals all the evils of the cook pot.

Dr. Stephanson, the discoverer of the white Esquimaux says the following about salt: "As a result of my experiences in the Arctic, I consider salt as a positive hindrance to live. I found its use absolutely eliminated from the dietary of the Esquimaux, who would rather submit to the ravages of starvation than to use food cured or seasoned with salt. Like tobacco, salt has conquered our taste and instinct, by the unnatural craving created by its indulgence as a stimulant, resulting in a habit difficult to break away from." Dr. Stephanson, describes the action upon himself and his followers as a narcotic poison.

Most housewives know that salt is fatal to chickens and canary birds as well as all other birds. Very often the cause of "chicken cholera", "gapes", and the like has been traced to the presence of salt—in large quantities—in food left over from the table.

In the human, salt hinders the digestion of albumen, by interfering with the secretion of gastric juice. Those who are liable to attacks of gout often find themselves entirely free from their trouble when abstaining wholly from salt, but suffer a relapse immediately, when salt is taken into the system. Inflammation of kidneys is greatly aggravated by the use of salt.

Over consumption of salt is largely responsible for eczema and other skin diseases. Its ill effects are especially apparent upon the kidneys, as upon those organs depends the ridding of the body of a poison, which can not be utilized. Dropsy, and certain form of heart disease are in many cases caused in whole, or in part, by the free use of salt. Many people become immune to colds, after they abandon the use of salt.

It is often said in the defense of salt, that animals resort to "salt licks." I know of a horse that chews tobacco and of many dogs that drink beer. It will always be found that the food on which the animals have been feeding is deficient in certain natural organic salts, perhaps owing to poverty of soil causing them in time to acquire unnatural taste.

Salt is a great cause of premature old age, it hardens the tissues, especially the arteries, (arterial sclerosis.)

Salt is an irritant, it produces irritating effects in the system, indicated by dryness of the throat, and acceleration of the pulse.

Salt is not taken up by the system. It is always expelled unchanged by the liver, kidneys, skin and all the other depurating organs.

Chlorine and sodium in their organic state are useful and necessary minerals. You can only get organic chlorine and sodium from Natural Foods, i. e. Unfired Foods.

Chlorine and Sodium in form of "Salt" is inorganic (Disorganized) and can not be assimilated by your system. Beware of it!

MILK

Mothers milk is the ideal food for babies, because it is natural. Natural milk NEVER comes in contact with the air.

Cow's milk is the ideal food for the calf with its four stomachs; it is a poor food for the human baby with only one stomach. Whenever the mother is unable to feed her baby, unfired nut milk, vegetable juices or fruit juices should be used instead of cow's milk.

Vegetables and fruit juices can safely be given to babies after the fourth day, they are very wholesome and since the milk of the "city mother" is in most cases deficient, these juices are valuable additions.

Pasteurization is for the purpose of keeping bad milk in a saleable condition and for no other purpose. Fear, excitement, bad food and unsanitary conditions of the stables affect the cow's milk and in turn the baby. Fruit or vegetable juices never have bad effects on the infant.

No animal will give milk naturally after weaning its young, unless made a milk factory of by humans.

Sterilized milk and cream put up in sanitary bottles, is handled by a milk driver with the same sterilized (?) hands he handles his horse and this milk bottle stands for several hours on a sterilized (?) back porch where sanitary (?) cats have access. How many people sterilize the necks of those sanitary milk and cream bottles, before pouring the milk into the pitcher for the break-feast table? Since the germ theory is only propaganda to inject fear and raise milk prices (on account of the high cost of sterilization,) these germs from the horse, the drivers hands the back-porch and the cats fortunately are doing no harm unless they get into a filthy diseased stomach where they find food to thrive.

In the Unfired diet we never use sweet milk or cream, because it forms tough and indigestible curds in the stomach. We "lemonize" the milk in order to prevent these curds, or we use buttermilk. Too much milk is not advisable.

Milk cures and milk diets are in vogue at present, but the results obtained are not lasting nor can they be called cures. If you are in a rundown condition you can very quickly put on weight by going on an exclusive milk diet. But weight is not Health.

When a patient is put on a milk diet, he is artificially fattened, like the farmer fattens his pigs. The diseased condition is covered with fat. As soon as the patient stops the fattening process the disease symptoms reappear; but the patient has left the sanitarium by this time and the doctors of the institution praise the wonderful results of the milk diet.

When you go on a Raw Food Cure, you lose weight, because you have to eliminate several pounds of diseased matter, then you build up gradually to your normal weight.

Butter is unnecessary in the unfired diet, because you get plenty of fats from your nuts, which should go with most of your meals.

Cottage Cheese is wholesome but be cautious in its use on account of its large contents of protein, which may harm you if your stomach is not in its very best state. Most of the other kinds of cheese should not be used because they contain salt; a very harmful mineral, which I will explain later.

"The other side of every cloud
Is bright and shining.
And so let's turn our clouds about
And always wear them inside out
To see the lining."

Too much reading causes constipation of the brain, independent thinking is the natural enema for a constipated brain.

Diarrhea of words is always associated with a constipated brain.

MENSTRUATION

The monthly menstrual flow is a natural and normal function in a woman; therefore the term "unwell," "sick," etc., should never be applied to this function unless you apply these terms to breathing, eating or the evacuation of the bowels.

The unfired diet tends to regulate the monthly flow. It usually cures too profuse flowing, and in general lessens the flow. When beginning the unfired diet it very often happens that a woman will stop flowing for a month or two, or miss every other month within four months, but as soon as the system has adjusted itself to the natural diet, the flow will be more regular and connected with little discomfort or pain.

Most of the women I know of experienced no more pain and the flow was greatly lessened after they began the unfired diet and some of the cases on record often were not even aware that they were flowing until they found material evidence of it.

Normal menstruation should never be connected with pain or discomfort. Live naturally, and your organs will function naturally every month instead having a monthly "sickness."

VENEREAL DISEASES!

This part of the book is printed in bold type, because I want you to read about a widespread condition, which is commonly carefully hidden.

Over 90 per cent of all men are suffering from Gonorrhea or Syphilis at one or another time of their life. These diseases are in most cases the effect of promiscuous sexual intercourse.

The majority of venereal diseases in the male are never cured; they are mostly suppressed through the use of drugs, dopes and serums.

Serums, salvarsan, "606," etc., never cured syphilis. Gonorrheal serum does not cure gonorrhea. These poisons only hide the diseases so they cannot be detected by unreliable tests like those commonly used in the laboratory, i. e. the Wassermann test for Syphilis or the Microscope for Gonorrhea,

In general the public takes too much stock in the different laboratory tests of the aforesaid kind. The Wasserraann test is positively useless because certain conditions of intoxication will show a "positive Wassermann," where there may be no syphilis present, while a syphilitic patient will often show a "negative Wasserman" simply because he partook of certain foods.

Gonorrhea is determined by the use of the microscope. When there are no more "gonococci" showing the disease is supposed to be cured; but the microscope and the human eye are very limited and particularly in this case, let me illustrate this.

A young man is suffering from gonorrhea; he is being treated by his medical doctor in the "regular" way, with corrosive injections, alkaline pills, and for good measure with gonorrheal serum. After a few weeks of this "radical" treatment the visible symptoms, pain, discharge, etc., disappear, Mr. M. D. is very careful; he will not declare his patient cured until he has carefully examined the urine etc., of his patient under the microscope. He finds no more gonococci or "bugs" and he is satisfied that the patient is cured.

The same young man gets married a year later. The young wife notices a discharge from her sex organs, she consults another lady friend and after being told that such a thing is "NOTHING" just the "Whites" she does not pay any more attention to this state, which seems to be a necessary evil connected with married life. The discharge is irregular, sometimes very profuse, and other times very scant, but always present.

Usually after the first child greater disorders connected with much pain are noticed, but this is blamed on the childbirth. The friends and neighbors say: "Since she had her child she is always ailing."

Things get worse and the wise man, the family physician, is consulted, and after careful examination, he finds that some part of the sex anatomy is diseased, and like a good (?) mechanic, he orders the diseased part taken out and thrown away (What would you do to your repairmen if he finds a broken part on your auto and he throws it away and tells you to run without it?)

"The lady needs an operation' If she does not know any better she will submit to the "mutilation' and after her first Mutilation she is a proud member of the great and ever growing society of crippled women, who have no more pleasure or purpose in life except to be operated on at intervals when their pocketbook permits it, and to relate the story of their terrible operations and the skill of their butcher to one another.

What was the cause of this woman's disease? A VENEREAL DISEASE — Gonorrhea. — The disease her young husband acquired while he was sowing his wild oats, the disease the wise doctor pronounced cured, because he could not find any more gonococci under the microscope on examination of the young man's discharges.

If gonococci were the disease producers of gonorrhea and not a germ which always happens to be present in gonorrheal pus, the young man would have been cured, but the doctor only eliminated the germ, he could not eliminate the disease with drugs or vaccines. Drugs and vaccines only suppress disease or change its appearance so it is impossible to be seen under the microscope.

Women!!! Do you know that eighty percent of all operations performed on you are caused by venereal diseases?

Women!! Do you understand that the tests used to determine the cure of venereal diseases are unreliable?

Women!! Do you know that 90 percent of all *men* are suffering at one time in their life from some venereal disease?

Women!! You cannot even blame these men, because most of them try their best to get cured, but the medical profession is unable to determine when they are cured, because they do not use reliable tests.

You need not get discouraged, because there is one test which will positively tell the presence of venereal disease, whether it is two hours or seventy-five years after infection, whether there are germs found or not, whether a Wasserman shows positive or negative. This test is called the BYO-DYNAMIC-CHROMATIC test

Dr. George Star White of Los Angeles, California is the inventor of this system of diagnosis. This test has been applied to over fifty thousand cases and always proven correct in every case.

Not only can hidden and suppressed venereal disease-conditions be revealed, but also cancer can be diagnosed before it is developing, so steps can be taken to avert this dreadful condition.

I shall give you a short description of the B. B C. Application of Diagnosis and its underlying principles.

Byo - Dynamic - Chromatic diagnosis means finding out what poison is in the system by the action of color on the living organism.

It is the only system of diagnosis known to science by which a man can be definitely determined to be free from disease toxin in his blood.

The currents of magnetism which keep a compass constantly pointing north have a definite effect on the human body. In a person free from disease poisons in his blood the effect is greater than in a person suffering from a systematic disease. This can be easily demonstrated scientifically.

Hold a magazine with its thin edge pointing north. Very few currents of magnetism will pass through it this way as you can plainly understand. However if you face the broad side of the magazine north then you will find that many currents pass through it. The same is true of the body. If the SIDE is faced north few currents cross the nerves of the body but if the FACE is faced north then many lines of nervous energy are crossed by these magnetic currents.

It is a law in electricity that if lines of magnetism cross other lines that induction takes place Therefore there would be little induction if the person were standing so that the SIDE faced the north but more induction would be produced when tie patient FACED north.

This induction changes the tention in the body enough to be noticeable if the proper technic is followed out. If the induction takes place the person is not suffering from any toxemia, such as syphilis, gonorrhea, malaria, cancer, and so on.

If this change in tension does not take place however then there is some toxemia or poison in the system which is affecting the man.

It is a scientific fact that all matter is electronic in its make-up and all matter is radio-active in a greater or lesser degree. In disease the emanations of energy from the body are different from the normal.

It is also a scientific fact that like vibrations neutralize each other. For the purpose of neutralizing these diseased energies we use colors of known vibration and by using one color after another we will find one which will allow the indication spoken of above to take place and when we do, we know that the patient is temporarily normalized and we know then what the disease is. We standardized the vibrations in the color screens used. (*)

Women, it is a duty to yourself and the coming race, your children, to be informed of the state of health of the man you marry, the father of your offspring. The B. D. C. test will give you this information; it is the only reliable test.

Young men and women, you can save yourself much suffering by being tested by the B. D. C. method before entering the state of marriage.

All venereal diseases CAN BE CURED, provided you use the natural method. Always consult a doctor who uses the B. D. C. Method of diagnosis and you can rest assured you are in good hands. Do not consider venereal disease filthier than any other disease, the time will come when men and women will all be ashamed to be sick and will then co-operate with nature's laws.

Progressive physicians all over the world are taking up the study of the B. D. C. method of diagnosis and are discarding unreliable laboratory tests. Time will not be far off when venereal diseases will be on the decrease instead of being on the increase like they are at present.

Unfired food cures venereal diseases. Systematic fasting, followed by a strict fruit—and herb— diet with plenty of sunshine and fresh air have been very successfully employed. But every case of venereal disease should be cured under the guidance of an experienced drugless doctor who employs all the latest methods of diagnosis as mentioned above.

---

* Description of the B. D. C. Method of Diagnosis by courtesy of Dr., J. W. Wigelsworth.

FOOD IN RELATION TO SEX

The strongest of all the bodily appetites of the natural instincts are the sexual functions. They are the most important source of health and happiness if performed normally and exercise the most beneficial influence on all mental and bodily functions. The want of gratification of the normal sexual instinct is the source of great moral and mental suffering, lessening the love of life and inducing sadness and despondency.

The foundations of all sexual feelings are healthy physiological functions. They are not sinful nor do they exist in opposition to all that is noble in man or woman. They are of the greatest importance for the welfare and happiness of the human race.

The participation of the opposite sexes in the sexual relation through the attraction of love is one of the most beautiful phenomenon of existence, and when properly conducted, is in no sense to be constructed as vulgar or disgusting, which religious ascetics have described as lust.

We should never regard our normal sexual feelings as something low, vile or lustful as theological morality has taught.

It is the sexual instinct which is the source of all that is pure and noble within the human race, despite the raving of immoral theological and other "moralists" (?) who attempt to suppress the normal activity of the functions of the human body, even, if it is done with the best intentions and with the belief that it qualifies the individual for the attainment of happiness in another life.

The old and foolish conception that this life is a valley of tears, that must be endured until we are transported to the seventh heaven of everlasting happiness, must be replaced by a more material one in which LIFE and not

"After Death" is regarded as our opportunity for growth and development and our immortality must consist in the contribution made by us to the sum total of human happiness.

If sex is to be regarded as an evidence of sinfulness, deserving only to be suppressed, stifled, and killed, in order that the divine spiritual elements or the better qualities belonging to human nature may become manifested in our life and conduct, then we have conclusive evidence that the creator made an unpardonable mistake and should have consulted some of the antiquated theologians, who are responsible for many of the erroneous ideas concerning the "baseness," "lowness" and "sinfulness" of this beautiful, psychic, and physical instinct.

Sex is that element with which one human being blesses another.

The world's strongest, greatest, most useful men and women are those, who are born with a strong, natural sex-desire, but they are not libertines.

Ascetics or puritans deserve no credit for being virtuous, for they really are not, as they are usually from birth born weak, devoid of the normal bodily appetites, and consequently they never had a single normal sexual desire to resist.

The sexual relation is only an incident in the marital union of two well-developed individuals and is one of the numerous ties which unite and hold husband and wife together.

The fundamental conditions of a happy marital union are comradeship, understanding, mutual interest, sympathy, loyalty, and all that contributes to the happiness, success and development of the entire personality.

Neither marriage licenses nor churches will create happiness for married people, safety for children or happy homes. Love alone can do this and where it is absent, a union is false and marriage is an unworthy oppression, which ruins character; and all prattle of infidelity is without inner, deeper import.

If the sexual act is the only tie that binds the marital relation, such a relationship is not love, but can only be compared with prostitution licensed by the church or state.

Such a relation is devoid of devotion, and thus the main element of sexual life is lacking. The sex-act which is being performed as the result of habit without love or sympathy, in response to the physiological demands of the animal nature, results in no gratification for one party and causing humilliation for the other. Sickness, suicide, divorce or the most unhappy state of existence is the consequence of such marriage relations, which are more the rule than the exception of our present day.

Where the fundamental conditions of love for a happy marital union enumerated above exist, and the individuals concerned are endowed with a vigorous sexual nature, sex may still become a menace to them unless guided and controlled by the mind.

The mind can only function properly when it is balanced. Stimulating (cooked) foods, unbalance the mind, in the same degree as they unbalance the stomach. Neither will know when they have enough.

Let me call your attention to the wide-spread fallacy that eggs eaten in large quantities will improve or strengthen a weakened sex power or cure impotency. They are simply stimulants, whipping your desire into action, but resulting in "no action." All "rich" foods will increase the desire for sex, but not the sexual powers.

Sex-stimulation, through food, has the same effect as the whip on a tired horse, keep on whipping the horse and you will kill it quicker. Artificially stimulated sex is controlled by the stimulant, instead by the mind, and it becomes the curse to humanity.

The sex act performed as the result of "food-stimulation" becomes an obsession which hounds the individual day and night and takes sole control of the mind. Every person of the opposite sex is looked upon by such individuals as an object for the gratification of their unnatural stimulated passions (lust).

Unfired food energizes but never stimulates sex. The sex of the individuals living on the unfired diet is more powerful and capable, but it is never in evidence unless called upon by them. Cooked food irritates the organs of reproductions, and the mind, causing physiological conditions, undermining the will, and making them slaves of passion.

"False ideas in regard to sex are the greatest cause of women being cold and unresponsive; the truth about sex will often change a Xantippe into a Venus."

Teach your children that every living thing, from man to insect is the result of the union between the sexes, the most sacred of all relations.

Parents who keep the truth about sex from their offspring are moral cowards and deserve the deepest contempt.

Nature is stronger than the church, sex is a product of nature, sex-suppressions a product of the church.

Innocence is something to be ashamed of. Do not confuse it with virtue; an innocent girl is an ignorant girl, she may be virtuous but she cannot be ignorant and stay virtuous.

THE ACTION OF THE HEART AND KIDNEYS IN THE UNFIRED DIET

I print the following letter I received some time ago. People are often alarmed when they find that after they live on the unfired diet that the quantity of the urine is greatly diminished.

Unfired Food contains less waste; therefore less urine (waste) has to be eliminated. Do not drink water in large quantities. The same water that washes wastes from those who eat cooked food would wash useful and essential elements from food and besides overwork the kidneys

Dr. D. writes: Have you noticed a slower heart on the unfired food diet? My heart was right at seventy-two per minute, and now is sixty per minute. I reason that the less poison to be excreted the more rest the heart can take, and as the unfired food throws less in the system to be excreted there is less for the heart to do. Anyway at this saving of twelve beats per minute in one year the heart will save 6,307,200 beats, or two months of rest more than it was getting in a year's time, and that means that it will last that much longer.

My specific gravity of urine has been at 1.000 to 1.004 on the unfired diet instead of 1.015 or 1.025 as given by the chemists, and of course the less of waste thrown off through the kidneys the lighter the urine will be.

Last Sunday we were invited out for dinner. The meal was about half and half fired and un-fired. That was the first fired meal I had eaten since the 11th day of April. In five or five a half hours after the meal the specific gravity of my urine was 1.002 and a sample that I had tested on Friday was 1.004, showing that the fired meal, contained enough of waste material to raise the specific gravity .008

points. And certainly no one would say that was because the fired diet contained more food value.

For the past three weeks or so my weight has been about the same. I am fuller in the face and think I have filled out a little but not enough to show much on the scales. I usually weigh less in the morning than in the evening. One night I weighed three pounds more than I did the next morning after the bowels had moved and the bladder had been emptied. I did not drink but just about two swallows of water as I was retiring, and did not drink before weighing. I calculate that the system disposed of about three pounds of waste material.

I am feeling better than I have for years and have no craving for fired food. Came home last Sunday and had my usual meal of unfired food and enjoyed it as much as ever.

THE STARVING BABIES OF AMERICA
By **DR. CARL LOEB**
(From Apyrtropher Magazine)

Much is written about the starving babies of the war-ridden countries of Europe which die by thousands on account of the lack of food, but little or nothing is known of the overfed children of the well-to-do in this country who are suffering from malnutrition, caused by ignorance, instead of poverty.

To be more exact; I mean the babies, which get the best of care, have a private nurse, are bathed so often, are fed by the clock, with certified, pasteurized or what other processed milk, and in addition are given some of the many so-called "scientifically" compounded baby-foods which give such wonderful results (in the advertising columns of the press).

Very likely you all have seen the results, some of these "healthy" looking infants. So "nice and fat," raised very much like the farmer raises his pigs, confined in a narrow space so they get as little as possible exercise, lots of rich food, plenty of sleep, and very little sunshine. Since the baby is a human product, it has many advantages in the way of acquiring fatty tissue, over the pig.

First of all it is born abnormally heavy, very often a monster of 9 to 10 pounds with a head of unusual proportions which would cause a normal mother considerable trouble at the time of delivery; but the modern woman, whose motherhood is one of the disadvantages of married life, and is considered a necessary evil, suffers more severely. The modern mother who dedicates and deforms her body to fit the latest styles, is a very suitable model for the display of the latest creations "de Paris," but very unfit for motherhood.

The pig mother did not eat for two and the little pig when born was nothing but skin and bones; while the mother of the baby was taught to eat for "two", and instead delivering a normal baby of skin and bones so to say, she had to go thru "the dangerous operation" instead through the "natural function" of childbirth.

The readers may get the idea, that they are reading the farm or stockgrower's magazine. Not so. The foregoing is only a little illustration in words. If I were an artist, I would paint a picture in colors to make you understand better.

Humanity is suffering very much from so-called " science" and traditional knowledge, brought down from our ancestors, and such "antiquated science" is even repeated in text books of medical schools.

Medical science gained and still gains most of its knowledge from the ABNORMAL in hospitals instead from the NORMAL human, or the still MORE NORMAL animal. The result of such investigation is used to make rules for the masses of the people.

Therefore, we need not be surprised about the wrong and foolish diet of the pregnant and nursing mothers which is in common use among the laity. When so-called authorities prescribe meat, eggs, bouillons, and even wine, beer, and whiskey for the expectant and nursing mother, instead prescribing foods rich in organic (organized) salts like green vegetables, fruits and nuts.

Meat, eggs, soups, etc., are commonly prescribed in cases of anemia, and also in general for pregnant women, in connection with useless and very harmful iron preparations, in the form of pills, and spurious beef iron and wine combinations.

All these different iron combinations, in form of pills, elixirs, etc., are faithfully swallowed in unbelievable quantities by the ignorant public, which is too lazy to think, and takes the contents of any selfish advertisement without a moment's hesitation, as long as the pill or tonic has the magic word "Dr." on the package or trade mark.

Our public is trained and "educated" by expert psychologists, who make it their business to study the weak points of the masses, so they are able to exploit them in the most efficient way, by means of advertising.

No wonder manufacturers of patent medicines, who sell their products at 25c to 50c per package to the public, and give the druggist a 30 percent discount, can spend millions of dollars per year for advertising to "educate" the public, while our public schools cannot even raise enough funds, to employ an adequate number of teachers and pay them a living wage.

All these inorganic iron preparations CAN NOT be assimilated by the human system, no more than the inorganic iron in the water containing rusty nails, which the allopaths of the old school used to prescribe. Therefore, all these preparations are useless and will not answer the purpose, they were intended for by the user; and besides are very harmful to the teeth and stomach.

Organic salts unorganized by chemical process, (nerve-foods, brain-foods, etc.), CAN NOT be taken up by the human system in tissue or cell construction.

The only salts which are useful are those contained in living plants, which change inorganic salts to organic salts. These are readily taken up by the human system, if they are not changed again by fire (cooking) to their inorganic state.

The allopaths claim that iron pills are absorbed. They are; but the iron is lodged between the cells and there accumulates as a poison, which shows prominently in the iris of the eye in the form of red marks. (See Dr. Lahn's Diagnosis from the Eye.)

The lack of organic lime (calcium) in the diet of the average mother, the lime which is necessary for the construction of the bones and teeth of the infant, manifests itself in the form of decaying teeth of the pregnant and nursing mother.

Meat does not contain any calcium. Eggs only contain calcium in the shell which is discarded. When the mother continues the egg and meat diet, the result soon shows on the child in form of rickets (rachitis.) Bowlegs are more often caused by rickets, and not by too early attempts to make the infant walk as is commonly believed by many mothers.

Let us consider the following and I will leave it to the readers to form their own conclusions.

The average woman during gestation eats for two. Why should a human being eat for two when cats and dogs do not eat for five or six?

The cow produces plenty of milk for its offspring by eating greens. So far no case of a cow is known, which needed beefsteak, eggs, several quarts of milk, rich soups, beer, wine, and whiskey per day to produce the necessary milk for its calf. Should we proud humans ignore the lesson from the cow? Yes, the cow is an animal, so is the human being, but is the fact that we are more highly developed animals a reason that we should show less common sense?

We are the only animals who put our young on the back. Imagine a little pony, monkey, duck, chicken, etc., put on its back by its mother, with its legs paddling the air! Don't laugh! You are one of the family. The joke is on you.

We bundle our little ones up, so they are unable to move, carefully protect their body from air and sunshine, and keep the sunlight from the sleeping infant.

The animal mother exercises its young from the day they are born. The human baby never regains the proportional strength it had at the time of birth. A new born baby can lift twice its own weight. How many athletes can perform this fete? Only because we ignore the natural laws, we make cripples out of our offspring. Are they not cripples if we destroy, thru neglect, 50 percent of the efficiency nature gave to them at birth, by willfully preventing them from using their limbs?

The foregoing statement is not a theory. Professor Banks, one of our co-workers, has startled the professional world by normal exercising and correct feeding, NOT TRAINING, of babies, so they were able to stand erect on the palm of his hand on the 7th day of their life. Babies were able to walk when they were $4\frac{1}{2}$ months old. The babies I mentioned before which are able to perform these seeming wonders, are not the offspring of great men and women. Most of them were inmates of a Chicago foundlings' home.

Prof. Banks promised to send us an article on his results and experience with infants. It will be the first article published on his work, so it is unnecessary for me to dwell on this subject any longer.

Mothers! After reading the foregoing, if you love your offspring, if you want to give them the only valuable treasure there is, a treasure, which no one can take from them, A SOUND MIND IN A SOUND BODY. Stop reading advertisements without thinking. Be careful what material you use to build the next house for a soul. Study nature. Do your OWN thinking. Don't pay a few pennies for some greedy person's thoughts and suggestions in a newspaper. The coming age is the age of the woman. Mothers, do not depend on the man. He has made a blunder of everything in the past. It is the woman now, who will have to protect her babies from disease and her grown children from wars.

Women, wake up, think and act! It is up to you to make man equal, and, if you will, superior to the animal, by studying the apyrtropher diet.

THE FIRST TELEGRAPH SYSTEM
A Little Story for Big Children.
By DR. CARL LOEB
(From Apyrtropher Magazine)

Many years before Morse invented telegraphy, Nature had equipped all her children with an elaborate telegraph system with receiving and sending stations in every part of the body of her creations.

These stations were discovered after hundreds of years by investigators of natural science and they called them nerves.

Each station is directly connected with a main station. The main station, called nerve center, receives constantly reports from all stations about the condition of the surrounding territory under its observation.

As long as there is no danger to the tissues which are controlled by the different stations, the owner of the wireless system is not aware of these safety stations or nerves. But as soon as something of importance happens, the owner is notified instantly so he can prevent any damage to his property.

Let me illustrate this: Mr. Jones sits in a crowded street car reading his newspaper. He is deeply interested in today's baseball score. While he is reading all stations are on the lookout except those which are busy reading the paper and conveying the thoughts to the central station of the whole, the brain. Enters a 200-lb. gentleman. He stumbles and lands with his size 10 foot and his additional weight on Mr. Jones' toe. Now let us see how the alarm works. As soon as Mr. Fatty steps on Mr. Jones' foot all the stations (nerves) report this fact to the main station (nerve centers). They in turn send the danger signal up the spinal cord to the central station, the brain. As soon as the brain receives the signal it classifies the sensation. Since it was a fat man and not a pretty member of the weaker sex the brain decides the sensation was disagreeable and instantly the alarm (pain) begins to operate.

As soon as the alarm is sounded, Mr. Jones' pulls back his foot. The nerves controlling the facial muscles change the interested expression into one which we call sour. If Mr. Jones is not able to control the alarm system at this point the alarm may spread to the vocal cords and a line of words may emanate from his mouth which are tabooed in a drawing room.

As soon as the fat gentleman excuses himself, the facial nerves operate into the opposite direction and turn the sour face into a smiling one. The nerves of the foot order a large blood supply from the veins to repair the damage done by the fat man, and Mr. Jones continues to read the baseball score.

In our days of civilization bells are most commonly used for the purpose of alarming and warning people of danger. Nature in its infinite wisdom did not supply its creations with bells because bells would be unhandy and cumbersome if they were attached to our body. Instead of bells Nature supplied us with a different kind of alarm which is more compact than a bell and does not take any space when not in use; but when it is in operation this alarm requires our whole attention. You are all well acquainted with Nature's perfect warning signal, PAIN. For all external disturbances this pain signal usually operates at the point of injury, but whenever there is an internal disturbance the alarm in the head operates. This operation is called a headache.

The above was an illustration of a minor accident to the person of Mr. Jones. Let us see how the system works on the inside in case of a major disorder.

Stagesetting: A regular Sunday dinner. The cook adds plenty of salt, pepper vinegar, etc., to the food in order to fool the sentries (nerves of the mouth). They are doped now and are unable to decide when the stomach has sufficient and the proper kind of food.

Mr. Jones eats, until he is full. He does not know when he has enough because the nerves are put out of commission by alcohol and condiments. The stomach has been overloaded and Mr. Jones gets tired. He goes to sleep.

The mixture in his stomach works while he sleeps. The illegal manufacture of alcohol begins in the stomach of Mr. Jones. He will very likely not be caught by any prohibition agent but Nature will get him every time.

He wakes up with the signal of autointoxication, a headache. If the other stations are in good working condition the stomach will eliminate the cause of the trouble by the way it came in. But Mr. Jones has so often abused his stomach that it got worn in time and it is unable to eliminate the MASH in the stomach, therefore the alarm sounds constantly in the form of a headache.

If Mr. Jones were one of the regular animals, like a dog or cat, he would go on a fast, or like some dogs which I watched eat some greens to clean out the stomach.

But Mr. Jones is one of the highest developed animals especially supplied by Nature with REASONING POWER.

Let us see how he uses his reasoning power. When the alarm sounds he simply goes to the next drug store and gets some dope which puts the alarm system out of order. Every drug store can supply this dope which will put the internal alarm out of order—just ask for a headache powder.

I think it would be a very good idea to apply Mr. Jones' method in general, for instance: Supply all policemen with cotton. In case of alarm have them stuff their ears with cotton so they are unable to hear. This would be a great saving to the municipalities in autos, motorcycles, etc. On account of the large size of the fire alarm bells, cotton would not be sufficient for the firemen and I would advise in this case to have them puncture their eardrums.

The foregoing sounds so ridiculous I am afraid some of the readers are getting insulted. I beg the pardon of those who have never taken a pill or dope to stop Nature's alarm, instead of stopping the cause. All the others have no reason to feel hurt.

Not all of you would have been as foolish as Mr. Jones who went to the druggist for dope to get rid of his headache. Some of you would have seen your doctor. There arts different varieties of doctors in the world. One finds the cause of the alarm (the headache) and removes the cause and not the alarm. The other disconnects the wires of the alarm system by giving dope.

If you were Mr. Jones, would you go to the Allopath who puts the wires of the alarm system out of order by giving dope, or would you go to the drugless doctor who treats the cause?

If you have a fire alarm on each corner of your city, and every time a person turns in an alarm you cut the wires, how long will your city last?

YOU ARE DOING THE SAME THING WHEN YOU TREAT DISEASE WITH DRUGS. You are cutting your life-wires but you are not extinguishing the fire which destroys you. After the allopath has cut all your wires and the alarm (all pain) stops, let the undertaker finish the job.

Poor Mr. Jones. If he would have been an Apyrtropher, he would have been unable to overeat or get a sour stomach, because he could not overeat on unfired food, nor will unfired food ferment in the stomach, but unfired food will cure a sour stomach. Had Mr. Jones taken some lettuce or other greens, with flaked nuts, he soon would have stopped the alarm (his headache) because the nuts neutralize the acid in the stomach and the greens sweep the intestines like a broom. Buttermilk is a still better neutralizing agent for a sour stomach than nuts, when used as a dressing on greens. But why have a sour stomach at all? Stomach trouble and constipation is the cause of over 95 per cent of all disease. It is impossible to suffer of stomach trouble or constipation when living on unfired food; but the great virtue of unfired food is not only disease prevention it also cures.

Dear Reader: "Don't you think it would be a good idea to investigate the Unfired Food Question and become your own doctor and master?"

DEAR READER:

I endeavored to give you a clear understanding of the laws and application of unfired dietetics, (Apyrtrophism.) I hope I succeeded.

Apyrtrophism is not a fad, nor a religion, and the people who belief in the efficacy of unfired food are not fanatics. They all came to that conclusion by carefully investigating the merits of unfired food. I wrote this little book to assist you in your investigation. It was not my desire to force my opinion on to you; if you are convinced of the superiority of the unfired diet, and you become an ardent Apyrtropher, be careful when giving your friends or strangers information about the natural diet.

You will be very enthusiastic when you experience the wonderful results of the unfired food on your own body, and you will want to help everybody; but remember advice is cheap, anything cheap is always considered—no good.— Do not give advice unless asked for. Let "them" coax you for information and they will appreciate it highly; but if you force your good will on to "them," they will not heed your advice and they will thank you for it by considering you a "Nut."

It takes investigation, knowledge and thinking to become an Apyrthropher. Remember only a minority is able to think. To become a fanatic adherent of a religious cult takes just the opposite, belief without seeing (investigating.)

Made in the USA